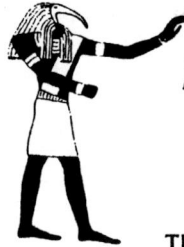

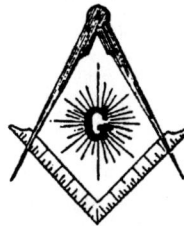

ZONE THERAPY

OR

RELIEVING PAIN AT HOME

BY

WM. H. FITZGERALD, M. D.

AND

EDWIN F. BOWERS, M. D.

Author of "Side Stepping Ill Health"
"Alcohol — Its Influence on Mind and Body," etc.

COLUMBUS, OHIO:
I. W. LONG, Publisher
1917

CONTENTS.

(3)

4   CONTENTS.

INTRODUCTION

THOUSANDS of lives are lost annually from diseases which could have been prevented. Hundreds of thousands, because of some preventable ailment, which partially or totally incapacitates them, are today living only a small part of their lives. Millions of dollars yearly are squandered on medicines, doctors and undertakers — much of which might have been saved by a right knowledge of the laws of health and hygiene.

Even among the comfortably situated, or even well-to-do, robust, vigorous health is the rarest of possessions. The most rugged-looking, on being closely and sympathetically catechised, will admit to a "touch of rheumatism"; a chronic stomach, liver, or kidney trouble; nervousness, headaches, neuralgia, constipation, or something that tends to prevent his attaining completest physical power and mental efficiency. And the weaker sex more than justify their descriptive adjective. For 80% of those not directly under a physician's care, or taking some medicine or form of treatment for something, should be.

Conditions are improving, however. There is a dawn of hope for humanity. For good health is being made a fetish. It is becoming a gospel — a gospel preached in schools, newspapers, magazines, churches and theatres. Accurate knowledge concerning sanitation, sexology, food, clothing, exercise, sleeping, resting, and all hygienic measures, is becoming more and more widely disseminated.

Humanity is awakening to the fact that sickness, in a large percentage of cases, is an error — of body and mind. Ignorance of the injurious effects of wrong foods, drinks, habits and methods is gradually being overcome.

Foremost among those engaged in educating the public away from paths of ignorance, and the disastrous consequences of this ignorance, is the medical fraternity. The noblest and most self-sacrificing profession on earth is the one most industriously engaged in sawing the branch between itself and the tree of Financial Gain. The doctor is the philanthropist most impressively employed in killing the geese that lay his golden eggs with one hand, while he cuts his pocket-book's jugular vein with the other.

For he catches and segregates — constructing prisons for them, if necessary — all cases, — or even suspected cases — of contagious disease, — disease which, if permitted to spread broadcast, would net him a horde of ducats.

He sees to it that no infectious disorders are imported into the country — the spreading of which would give him much practice. He traces every typhoid case to its ultimate dirty barn, or infected water supply, and counts that day well spent whose low declining sun has seen him stamp out a possible typhoid epidemic at its source

He vaccinates all — willing and unwilling — lest he be kept horribly busy attending a huge army of small-pox patients.

He instructs gluttons, and others, as to the grave dangers of overeating, or of eating the right food at the wrong time.

He teaches mothers to sterilize their babies' bottles, and thereby keep the bugs of war at bay.

He thunders against exposure, against spitting in or on public places; he has Health Ordinances passed, covering every conceivable method whereby disease might develop.

Untiringly and without intermission — except during a few of the worst blizzards — he inculcates the doctrines of flies, in their relation to fingers and filth, and hurls Phillipics against mosquitoes, ticks, and the insect world generally — not forgetting bed-bugs, lice, and other disease-breeding vermin.

He extols the benefits of bathing, the rich rewards of fresh air, exercise, and the relief of constipation.

In fact, he takes pride in doing all that within him lies, in order to teach the world to do without him.

Thanks to doctors, we are learning about plumbing and posture, mastication and measles, outdoors, deep breathing, poisons and poise. We are finding out what bad teeth do to good health, how to work, play and sleep so as to get the greatest physical good from each.

We are warned against overweight, alcohol, common colds and tobacco, and the evil possibilities in marrying one's cousin — or some one else's cousin who has, or has had, syphilis, feeble-mindedness, a drunken ancestry, epilepsy, or some tendency to "hark back" and "revert to type" — as did Mendel's beans, or the black Andalusian pullets.

The subject of life and health conservation is "in the air." Only recently a president of the American Medical Association made this theme the subject of his inaugural address. Hardly a medical journal but has one or more articles devoted to it in each issue. We are being specifically instructed in how to avoid disease.

Now, however, we are to learn how, in many instances, diseases, many of them most grave and life-shortening, may be cured. This, by measures which conflict with no other form of treatment, and so simple as almost to appear ridiculous. For Dr. William H. FitzGerald, the discoverer of zone therapy, is to tell us how he instructs his patients, under his guidance and direction, to cure themselves.

Dr. FitzGerald's position is one that commands respect. He is a graduate of the University of Vermont, and spent two and a half years in the Boston City Hospital. He served two years in the Central London Nose and Throat Hospital. For a like period he was in Vienna, where he was assistant to Professor Politzer and Professor Otto Chiari, who are known wherever medical text-books are read.

For several years Dr. FitzGerald has been the senior nose and throat surgeon of St. Francis Hospital in Hartford, and is an active member of most of the American medical societies.

I have known Dr. FitzGerald for many years. He is able and honest, a skillful and competent surgeon, and a student. No matter how foolish, how ridiculous his methods may seem, they are most decidedly not the vaporings of a dreamer or a charlatan. They are the calmly digested findings of a trained scientific mind.

And so Dr. FitzGerald is to give us specific

details of one of the most wonderful and perplex-
ing things connected with the art of medicine.
This, because a physician's premise is to teach —
as well as heal.   Because publicity concerning
the prevention and cure of disease is a duty he
owes mankind: not as an altruist, but as a human
being.

EDWIN F. BOWERS, M. D.

Sept. 1, 1916.

PUBLISHERS' NOTE.

THE chapters comprising this book were first published as special articles in the "Associated Sunday Magazines", and "Every Week". Accompanying the introductory article was this comment by Mr. Bruce Barton, the able and critical editor of these Magazines. It explains itself:

"For almost a year Dr. Bowers has been urging me to publish this article on Dr. Fitz-Gerald's remarkable system of healing, known as zone therapy. Frankly, I could not believe what was claimed for zone therapy, nor did I think that we could get magazine readers to believe it. Finally, a few months ago, I went to Hartford unannounced, and spent a day in Dr. Fitz-Gerald's offices. I saw patients who had been cured of goiter; I saw throat and ear troubles immediately relieved by zone therapy; I saw a nasal operation performed without any anesthetic whatever; and — in a dentist's office — teeth extracted without any anesthetic except the analgesic influence of zone therapy. Afterward I wrote to about fifty practising physicians in

(11)

various parts of the country who have heard of zone therapy and are using it for the relief of all kinds of cases, even to allay the pains of childbirth. Their letters are on file in my office.

This first article will be followed by a number of others in which Dr. Bowers will explain the application of zone therapy to the various common ailments. I anticipate criticism regarding these articles from two sources: first, from a small percentage of physicians; second, from people who will attempt to use zone therapy without success. We have considered this criticism in advance, and are prepared to disregard it. If the articles serve to reduce the sufferings of people in dentists' chairs even ten per cent., if they will help in even the slightest way to relieve the common pains of every-day life, they will be amply justified.

We do not know the full explanation of zone therapy; but we do know that a great many people have been helped by it, and that nobody can possibly be harmed."

THE EDITOR.

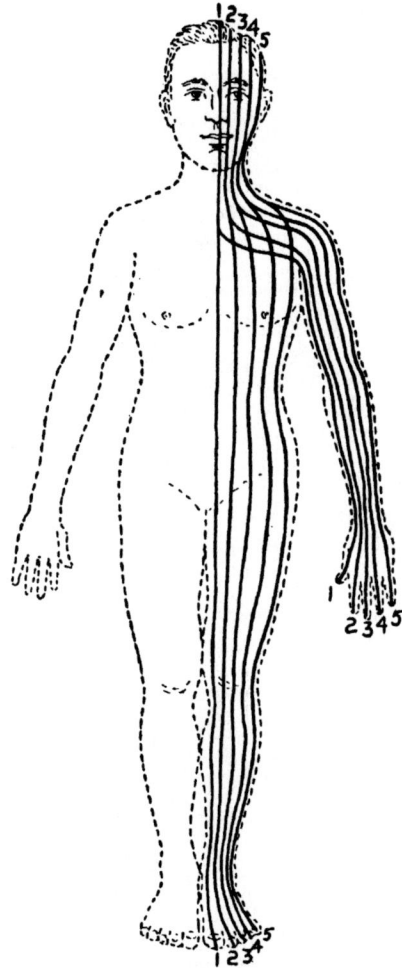

Diagram of **Anterior Zones** on one side of the body.

Both right and left sides of the body are the same.

Each numbered line represents the **center** of its respective zone on the anterior part of the body.

The tongue, hard and soft palate, posterior wall of the naso-pharynx and oropharynx, and the generative organs are in ten zones, five on each side of the median line.

The middle ear is in Zone 4.

The eustachian tube and middle ear combined are in Zones 3 and 4.

The upper surface of the tongue is in the anterior zones.

The teeth are in the respective zones as indicated by passing a line antero-posteriorly thru the respective zones.

The viscera are in the zones as represented by a line passed antero-posteriorly thru the respective zones.

FIG. 1.

(13)

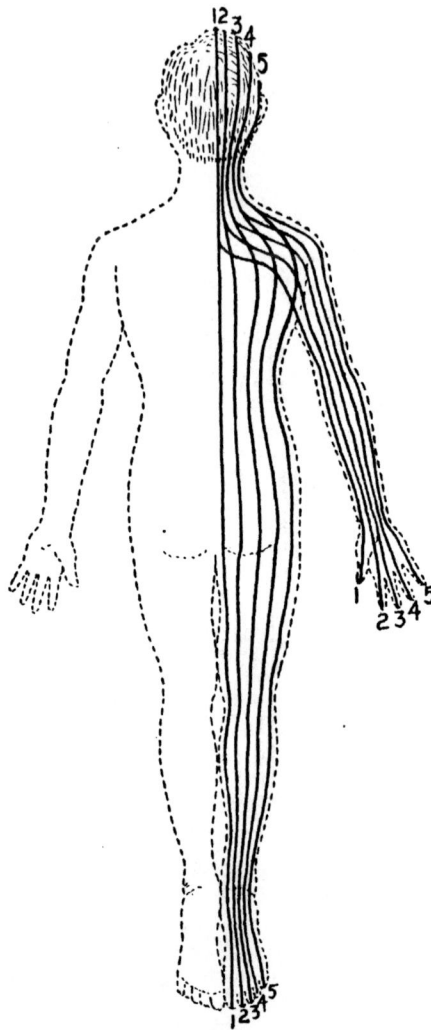

Diagram of **Posterior Zones** on one side of the body.

Both right and left sides of the body are the same.

Each numbered line represents the **center** of its respective zone on the posterior part of the body.

The under surface of the tongue is in the posterior zone.

FIG. 2. — Posterior view, illustrating individual zones. It will be observed that what is commonly called the back of the hand is really the front of that member, whereas the palm of the hand corresponds to the sole of the foot.

(14)

CHAPTER I.

NO illustrator would ever think of drawing a picture of a boy with a green-apple colic, unless he represented that boy with both hands clasped fervently over the seat of war. Nor would he picture a pain anywhere else, without showing the attempts made to relieve this pain. For no one would believe his illustrations, if he omitted these details.

Now, while we know the fact of pain relief, through laying on of the hands, or by kindred measures, we know only a part of its reason for operation. There are several of these. They are, first, the soothing influence of animal magnetism, experienced when we tenderly, if not lovingly, rub the bump, accumulated in the dark of the moon, by collision with a tall brunette side-board, or a door carelessly left ajar. It does soothe. This we know.

Next, the manipulation of the hand over the injured place tends to prevent a condition of venous stasis — a state in which the injured surface veins dam back the flow of blood, and produce that lurid discoloration known euphoneously as "black and blue."

Also, pressure applied over the seat of injury produces what Dr. George W. Crile, of Cleveland, calls "blocked shock," or "nerve block," which means that by pressing on the nerves running from the injured part to the brain area we inhibit or prevent the transmission to the brain the knowledge of injury. In other words, the hurt place can't tell the central telegraph station anything about the accident, because the wires are down.

Dr. Crile, and surgeons generally, now utilize this knowledge to prevent shock during operations, by injecting cocain, or some anesthetic solution around the course of the nerve trunk leading from the place to be operated upon to the brain.

But there is yet another reason, which we have found out only yesterday. And this is zone analgesia. Pressure over any bony eminence injured, or pressure applied upon the zones corresponding to the location of the injury, will tend to relieve pain.

And not only will it relieve pain, but if the pressure is strong enough and long enough it will frequently produce an analgesia, or insensibility to pain, or even a condition of anesthesia

— in which minor surgical operations may be successfully done.

This, of course, is not an infallible or invariable result. Specialists in zone therapy have found pressure effective in obliterating sensation in about 65% of cases; while it will deaden pain, or make it more bearable, in about 80%.

In the hands of many who have tried these methods the percentage often is much lower — because they haven't learned how to apply it. For if the operator doesn't "hit" the proper areas or focal points he misses them completely — and also misses results.

In attempting the relief of pain by "working" from the fingers it should also be emphasized that it makes a difference, too, whether the upper and lower or the side surfaces of the joint are pressed. A physician experimenting with the method was ready to condemn it because he was unable to relieve a patient who complained of rheumatic pains which centered on the outer side of the ankle-bone. The doctor grasped the second joint of the patient's right little finger and pressed firmly for a minute on the top and bottom of the joint. (See Fig. 3.) The pain persisted, and the doctor jeered at the method.

A disciple of zone therapy smiled, and suggested that while the doctor had the right finger,

2

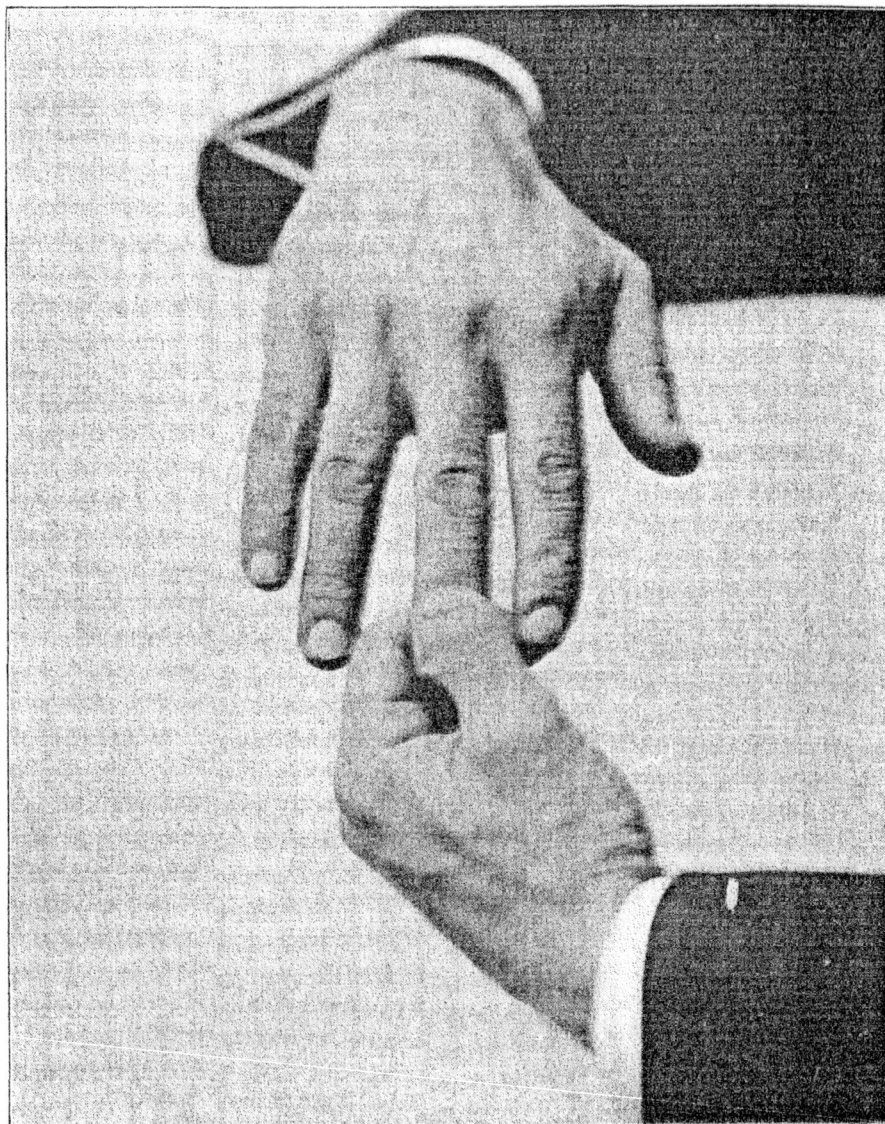

FIG. 3. — Illustrating method of applying anterior and posterior pressure to the finger joint.

he had the right finger in the wrong grip. The doctor was advised to press the sides of the finger (See Fig. 4), instead of the top and bottom. This was done, and the pain disappeared in two minutes.

This pressure therapy has an advantage over any other method of pain relief, inasmuch as it has been proved that, in contradistinction to opiates, when zone pressure relieves pain it likewise tends to remove the cause of the pain, no matter where this cause originates. And this in conditions where seemingly one would not expect to secure any therapeutic, or curative, results.

For instance, I recall a case of breast tumor, with two fairly good-sized nodes, as large as horse chestnuts. This lady had made arrangements to be operated upon by a prominent surgeon in Hartford, but had postponed her operation a few weeks on account of the holidays.

Meantime she had been instructed to make pressures with a tongue depressor and with elastic bands (See Figures 17 and 5), for the relief of the breast pain — which relief, by the way, was quite complete. After a few weeks, this lady returned to her surgeon for further examination and to complete arrangements for operation. Upon examining, however, the sur-

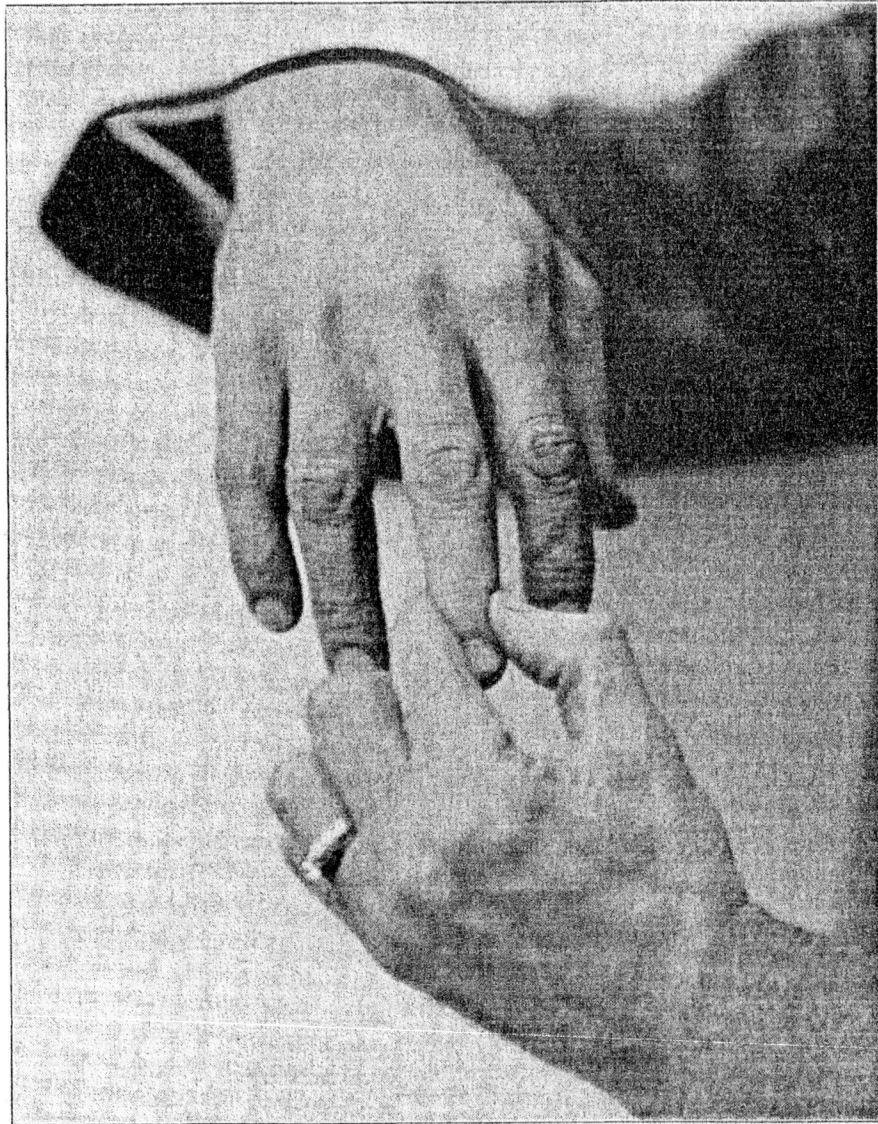

FIG. 4. Illustrating method of applying lateral pressure to the finger joint.

geon found the growth so reduced in size that he expressed himself as unwilling to operate, as he saw no necessity for operating. The tumor has since completely disappeared — under these tongue pressure treatments. This patient, and the name of the surgeon who saw her "before and after," are at the disposal of any physician who may regard this plain unvarnished tale as an old wives' chronicle.

A small uterine fibroid made a similar happy exit, as a result of pressures made on the floor of the mouth, directly under the center of the tongue. This patient next made a regular practice of squeezing the joints of her thumb, first and second finger, whenever she had nothing else important to do. And the result infinitely more than justified the means.

Lymphatic enlargements, as painful glands in the neck, arm-pits, or groin, yield even more rapidly to this zone pressure than do tumors. And while no claims are made to the effect that cancer can be cured by zone therapy, yet there are many cases in which pain has been completely relieved, and the patients freed from the further necessity of resorting to opiates. And in a few cases the growths have also entirely disappeared.

The growth of interest in this work is most

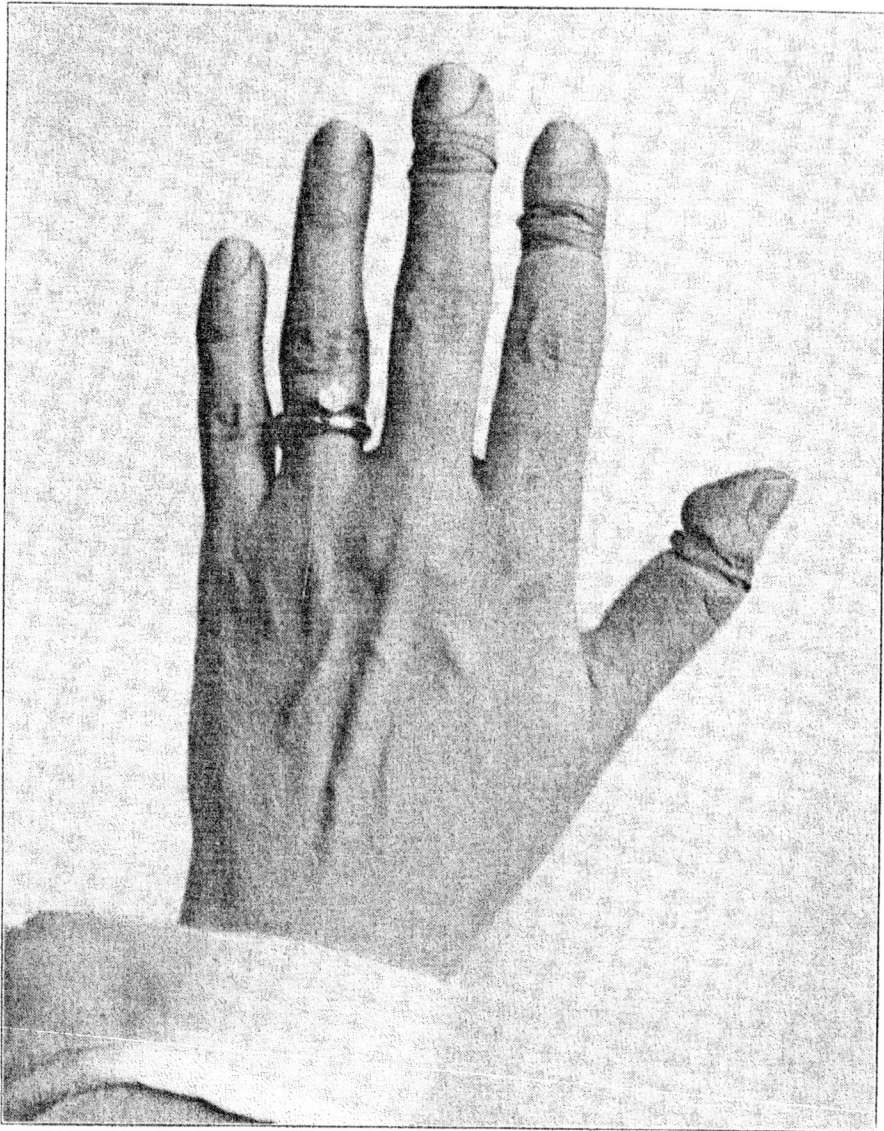

FIG. 5. — Showing method of "rubber-banding" the fingers for trouble
in the first, second and third zones.

encouraging. Dr. FitzGerald and other physicians using zone therapy in their practice, have had scores of letters from patients they have never even seen, but who have written, expressing their appreciation for the relief secured through instructions from some of their patients, or through following out some suggestion from my articles in the magazines.

I have reason to believe that there are now upwards of two hundred physicians, osteopaths and dentists, using these methods every day, with complete satisfaction to themselves and to their patients.

And the number of laymen, and especially laywomen, who are preaching the doctrine in their own households, and among their circle of friends, must be legion. The adoption of the method is attended with absolutely no danger or disagreeable results, and may be the means of lengthening short lives and making good health catching. I, for one, hope that the numbers of those who may be inclined to learn and practice these methods upon themselves and upon the members of their families may ever increase and multiply. For this is a big idea, and a helpful one. Therefore, the more who make it their own the better for the human race. We shall now let Dr. FitzGerald continue the argument.

CHAPTER II.

THAT ACHING HEAD.

THE next time you have a headache, instead of attempting to paralyze the nerves of sensation with an opiate, or a coal tar "pain-deadener," push the headache out through the top of the head. It's surprisingly easy.

It merely requires that you press your thumb — or, better still, some smooth, broad metal surface (See Fig. 6), as the end of a knife-handle — firmly against the roof of the mouth, as nearly as possible under the battleground — and hold it there for from three to five minutes — by the watch. It may be necessary, if the ache is extensive, to shift the position of the thumb or metal "applicator" so as to "cover" completely the area that aches.

Headaches and neuralgias, of purely nervous origin, not due to poison from toxic absorption from the bowels, or to constipation, or alcoholism, tumors, eye-strain, or some specific organic cause, usually subside under this pressure within a few minutes.

'Tis as easy as lying. Many patients cure

(24)

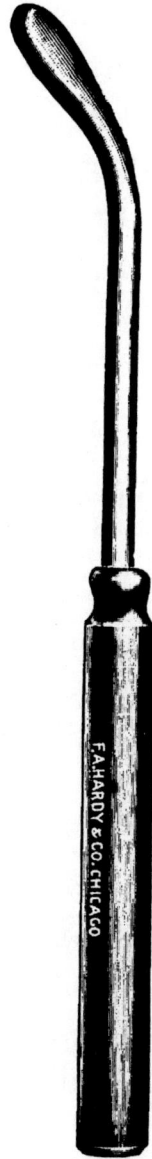

FIG. 6.—Palate-pressor Electrode may be used with or without electricity.

their own or their friend's and relative's headaches or neuralgic attacks in this manner. In
their own headaches they use their right or left
thumb — depending upon whether they are right
or left-handed. In treating others, they use the
first and second fingers, pressing firmly under
the seat of pain.

Their "points of attack" may extend from the
roots of the front teeth — for a frontal headache — to the junction of the hard and soft
palate — for a pain in the back of the head. Or
from the roots of the right upper molars to those
of the upper left molars, if the pain be in the
region of the temples or the side of the head.

Only temporary results should be expected —
or even complete failure — if the pain is due to
costiveness, eye-strain, or some persistent organic
condition — although even here the severity of
the attack can usually be modified.

In those headaches excited by dental operations relief can almost invariably be secured.
Dr. Thomas J. Ryan of New York, and others
familiar with zone therapy (the science of relieving pain and curing disease by pressures in
the various "zones" affected by pain or disease),
almost uniformly cure headaches or neuralgias
in their patients in this manner. In medical
practice the results are even more miraculous.

One of the worst cases yet treated by zone therapy was that of a lady who had suffered from persistent headache for more than three years. She had been to all the most prominent nerve specialists in the East, and had also consulted several European experts. Her heart was in a very dangerous condition, owing to the amount of antipyrin and other headache powders she had taken.

Her pain was located most generally in the forehead, and during the height of the attacks extended up as far as the top of the head.

It was not relieved by sleep — indeed, it was worse, if anything, after such poor and inadequate sleep as she was able to get. This fact eliminated eye-strain as a cause, for eye-strain headaches are almost invariably better after a night's rest.

Every organ in the body had received a most thorough overhauling, and still those headaches held the fort. So the diagnoses settled down into "pain habit."

Christian Science, magnetic healing, faith cure, and most of the modern medical fads had all been tried, without success. She was on the verge of suicidal melancholia.

The afternoon I first saw her she was almost in hysteria — her pain was so acute. For when telephoning for her appointment she had been told not to take any opiates — as they might "mask the symptoms," and confuse the diagnosis.

Without stopping to question her, I washed my hands in an antiseptic solution, placed the tips of the first and second fingers of my right hand close against the roots of her incisor, or front teeth, held her head rigidly with the left hand, and pressed firmly for two minutes. I then moved my finger tips an inch further back on the hard palate, and repeated the pressure for another two minutes.

Releasing her, I stepped back, much as an artist might, in viewing a piece of work that pleases him. That I was justified in so doing was proved by the fact that, for the first time in three years, except when under the complete influence of an opiate, this lady was absolutely free from pain.

I instructed her husband, who accompanied her, just where to make the proper pressures when the pain returned, and within a week had a report from him that there were now no further attacks of the neuralgic headaches. This relief has persisted for more than a year.

Headaches frequently respond to pressures exerted over the joints on the thumb or fingers, or sometimes it may be necessary to "attack" it from the inside of the nose, or from some other point of vantage in the zone affected.

As an illustration of how pain can be squeezed out of the head through the fingers, a typical case, reported by Dr. George Starr White, of Los Angeles, California, may be helpful.

A lady suffered from a very severe headache on the top of her head, which had persisted for more than three weeks. She had consulted several doctors, who had given her "coal tars," opiates, and hypodermics, but the relief was only temporary.

Dr. White told her nothing of what was contemplated, but took hold of her hands, and began firmly pressing on the first, second and third fingers — the pain being diffused over the frontal regions — at the same time engaging her in conversation concerning her condition.

After about three minutes he asked her if she would locate with her hand just where the pain was. She hesitated, looked up, and said, "Do you use mental therapy?" Then, after blinking perplexedly for half a minute, she added: "For the first time in three weeks, except when I've been under the influence of narcotics, the pain is entirely gone."

Dr. White told her to have someone repeat these finger pressures, at the same time emphasizing that if she failed to get relief from this method to come back.   He has not seen her since.

But the same condition in the same patient may not be cleared up from the same point every time.   For instance, if the pain is in the second zone of the forehead, at one time we may stop it by "attacking" the forefinger.   The next time, however, pressure upon that finger might not have the slightest effect, and we would have to go to the tongue or the roof of the mouth to get results.   Another time we might be successful only from the nose — or by pressing the teeth of an aluminum comb on the skull, above or below the seat of pain — and so on.

Now, physicians have for many years, been consistently teaching our patients and the public how not to get sick.   Why not carry this teaching to its only logical conclusion, and teach them how, by perfectly safe and harmless means, they may, if sick, cure themselves of their minor ailments?

It would add marvelously to the sum total of health, happiness, and economic efficiency if all headaches, for instance, which could be cured by zone therapy were cured and kept cured — by spreading the knowledge of how to keep them cured.

We feel certain also that the medical profession, as soon as it is generally informed concerning zone therapy, will eagerly welcome the opportunity to promulgate the advantages of a safe and harmless method of relieving headache and pain. And also of doing away with the necessity for longer resorting to dangerous antipyrin or phenacetin tablets and powders. This is a crusade worthy of their highest altruism and noblest self-sacrifice.

CHAPTER III.

CURING GOITRE WITH A PROBE.

ONE of the most obstinate disorders that afflict humanity — and one which seems to be rapidly on the increase — is goitre. Goitre is a general condition, in which the thyroid gland becomes progressively enlarged, producing an unsightly swelling low down on the front of the neck.

Associated with this swelling — whether as a cause or as an effect no one knows for a certainty — is a distressing state of nervousness, apprehension, and general discomfort.

Frequently the case becomes "exopthalmic" in type, running a pulse of 150 or more to the minute, and later developing irregularities in the heart's action. In this form there is also a marked protrusion of the eye-balls, from prespressure behind the globes of the eye, due to disturbances in the local circulation.

Many causes have been assigned for goitre, but no one knows for certain which is the correct one. Because of its prevalence in Switzerland and in other mountainous regions, where the inhabitants are obliged to depend upon water which was originally snow for their drinking supply, it was thought that the condition arose as a result of the lack of lime and other mineral salts ordinarily found in water which had been more intimately in contact with the earth. Yet the feeding of these mineral salts to those afflicted with goitre made no appreciable difference in the condition of these patients.

Other observers have ascribed goitre to the influence of the nervous tension, under which we live in this era of break-your-neck-to-get-there-and-do-it. Others locate the seat of this disease in the brain itself, in the blood vessels, and in the blood; others, who favor the so-called "mechanical theory," ascribe the symptoms to compression by an enlarged thyroid gland of the nerves and vessels in the neck, although they neglect to tell us how the gland became enlarged, in the first place.

Many authorities claim that the trouble originates most frequently as a result of eye strain. They insist that the visual centres, using as they do, one-third of all the brain energy, are overworked, in our intensive modern life, and react upon the body to produce the toxins of fatigue. The thyroid body, one of whose functions it is to secrete a product which tends to neutralize these

3

toxins, works overtime on the job, and not knowing when to quit, keeps right on working—with the result that the system is overcharged with thyroid extract. This thyroidism, as it is called, ultimately produces the goitrous symptoms.

Other clinicians contend that the disease is of microbic origin — which is quite unlikely — because when the glands have been brought to the autopsy table and the pathological laboratory, microbes have not been found in quantity sufficient to cause these grave symptoms.

But what interests and discourages those afflicted most is that if the cause is known, the successful treatment is even more unknown.

Medical men have treated these conditions on the general supposition that there was either too much or not enough thyroid extract secreted and discharged into the circulation by the thyroid gland.

So they gave thyroid tablets, made from the dried and pulverized glands of sheep. If these diminished the intensity of the symptoms, the doctors knew that the gland was deficient in its functioning powers, and that furnishing an additional supply from the glands of our woolly brothers would tend to restore the thyroid deficiency in us.

If, on the other hand, thyroid medication ag-

gravated the condition, the physicians figured
that the patient already had more thyroid substance than he knew what to do with. Hence
they administered iodine in some of its combina-
tions — generally as iodide of potash — in order
to bring about a more active condition of the
glandular system, and assist in the elimination
of this extra thyroid secretion.

If the gland still grew, and the symptoms became worse, there remained the alternative of
ligating or "tying off" the lobes, in order to
diminish the secreting power of the organ. Or,
more radical, yet hardly more generally effective,
an operation was made — extirpating (cutting
out) a considerable portion of the body of the
thyroid.

This, as may be imagined, is a very serious
operation, and fraught with considerable danger.
Not so much from the operation itself, as from
the consequences of the operation upon the psychological and mental condition of the patient.
Not infrequently the entire nature and disposi-
tion of an individual may be changed by the
apparently simple procedure of removing a few
cubic inches, or less, of tissue.

So, on the whole, goitre has been a bugbear—
most unsatisfactory from every angle. Yet,
with the proper application of the principles of

zone therapy, goitre—including the most advanced forms of exopthalmic—is one of the many conditions we are most certain of curing.

Almost from the first treatment, the feeling of suffocation, the distressing nervous symptoms and the pulse rate are favorably influenced. In from two to eight months the "pop eye" and the swollen gland are progressively reduced to normal.

Up to this writing, I have had more than thirty cases, every one of which, with two exceptions, have been cured and discharged, or are well on the way towards a cure. The tape measure shows that in some of these patients the swelling decreased three inches in as many weeks. One very responsive case was reduced from $14\frac{1}{2}$ to 13 inches in less than three days' treatment. The photographs accompanying this chapter speak for themselves. (See Figures 7 and 8.) There is no possibility of doubting the actual accomplishments of this method in the face of these visual demonstrations. And, as with all matters detailed in these pages, the original patients and data may be seen by any medical man who is fairly interested.

The explanation for the non-relief of the two cases which did not improve under treatment is simple—and very conclusive to those familiar

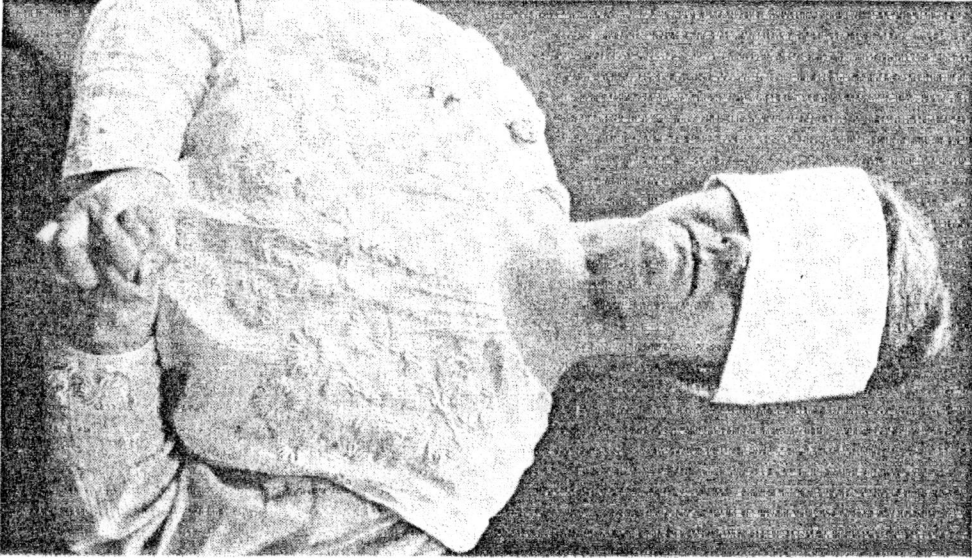

FIG. 7.

(See over)

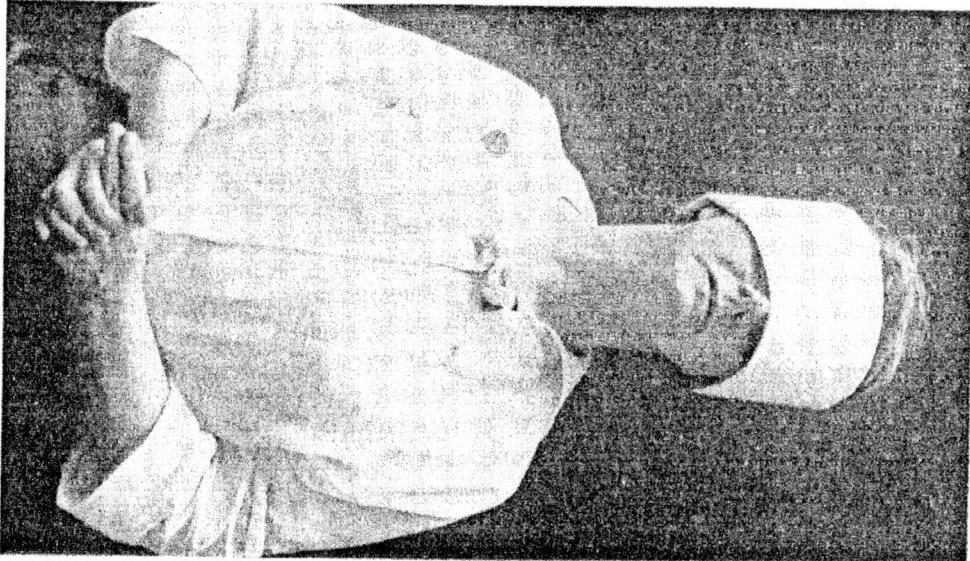

FIG. 8.

FIGS. 7 and 8.—Photographs of patient from New Hampshire, who consulted me April 1st, 1914, with well-marked bilateral goiter of two years' standing. Patient had had constant pressure and frequently pain over sternum for three months, but responded quickly to distal pressures, and was agreeably surprised to learn that the pain and discomfort would disappear for hours after pressure as depicted in illustration. Twice daily the patient exerted pressure on the posterior wall of the epipharynx via the nostrils with a cotton-wound applicator moistened with spirits of camphor—for its antiseptic effect merely.

Patient returned to New Hampshire the first of May, after one month treatment, or fifteen visits, considerably benefited. The growth had entirely disappeared by the middle of June. The last photograph was taken in Hartford, July 1st. Pressure through the thumbs and index and middle fingers of both hands, (inasmuch as only three zones on a side were involved), and pressure on the posterior walls of the epipharynx with metal applicator alternately, which she continued at home, was the only treatment she received.

with the method and its workings. One of these two non-benefited cases refused to carry out her "home treatment". The other was a patient suffering from an uterine tumor. This produced a pathological condition in the goitre zone. Hence the goitre would not yield until all other conditions influencing this zone were removed. I sent this lady to a gynecologist and it is quite certain that, after this tumor is removed, she will, under appropriate treatment, entirely recover from her goitre.

Dr. Reid Kellogg and Dr. Thomas Mournighan of Providence, R. I., Dr. George Starr White of Los Angeles, Dr. Plank of Kansas City, and a number of other medical men, have reported that they have the same uniformly favorable results in treating goitre that we have here.

Dr. Kellogg has had a dozen cases, all of which have been, or are being, cured. It is interesting to note that one of his cases, also, a lady suffering from a slight erosion of the neck of the womb, made no progress until this condition was cleared up by proper local treatment.

Dr. Mournighan has also reported on fifteen cases — eight of which were of the exopthalmic variety — all improving or discharged as recovered.

In treating goitre by zone therapy a thin probe, (See Fig. 9), the point of which is wrapped in cotton dipped in a little alcohol, spirits of camphor or camphor water (these seem to increase the "impulse") is passed through the nostrils to the posterior or back wall of the pharynx. Pressure is made in various spots "low down" on this wall (a little practice will soon determine almost the exact "spot" to probe), until a definite sen-

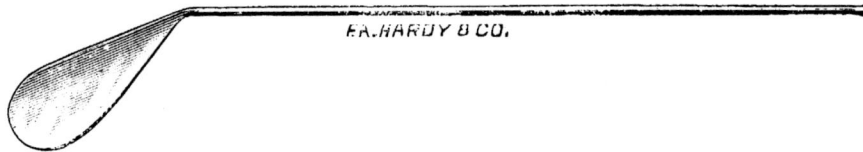

FA.HARDY & CO.

FIG. 9. — Special type of nasal probe used for attacking the posterior wall of the nasopharynx.

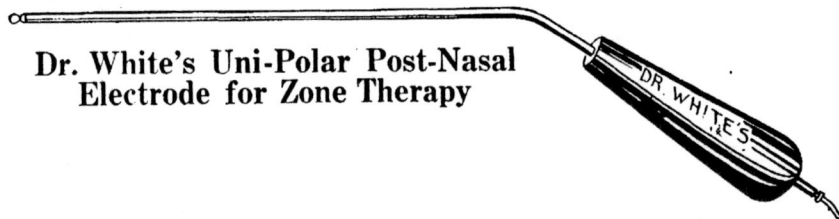

Dr. White's Uni-Polar Post-Nasal
Electrode for Zone Therapy

FIG. 10. — Dr. White's Uni-Polar Post-Nasal Electrode for Zone Therapy. May be used with or without electricity.

sation is felt in the region of the goitre. Sometimes this is "metallic". Or it may be a sensation of cold, or tickling, or like an electric current, or else a mild pain.

This pressure is held for several minutes — repeated three of four times daily. It can be done just as well by the patient himself, if he has the courage to hurt himself a trifle. In addition to the treatment on the pharyngeal wall, pressures may be made upon the joints of the thumb, first and second fingers, as shown in Figures 3 and 4. Or, if the goitre is a very broad one, and extends over into the fourth zone, the ring finger must also be employed. A moderately tight rubber band, worn upon these fingers for ten or fifteen minutes, (see Fig. 5), three or four times daily, will also help. Rubber bands may also be worn with benefit upon the toes governing the zones involved. But the treatment must be persistent. It must be the intent to keep the goitre zone "quieted," never allowing it, except during sleep, to come completely out of the influence of the pressure. And even during sleep in aggravated cases, moderate pressure should be continued.

I would especially emphasize the importance of seeing that the teeth are put in a perfect condition before attempting the cure of any case of goitre. For there is no doubt that the evil influence of bad teeth is not, by any means, confined to the throat and tonsils, as many observers contend. Indeed, I do not recall having ever seen a goitre case in which there was not something wrong with the teeth. I therefore make a routine practice of sending all goitre patients to their dentists for a thorough overhauling of their teeth when commencing treatment.

Also, it may be interesting here to note that if the theory of eye strain causation of goitre is true—and it seems quite likely that, in many cases, it may be — pressure therapy may logically be looked for to give satisfactory results. For the effects of eye strain can undoubtedly be relieved by pressure exerted on the first and second fingers, as we shall show in the next chapter.

So one of the most puzzling and unsatisfactory conditions with which physicians have had to deal can now be said to be almost invariably curable. And the only instruments we need to operate these grave conditions are a straight steel probe, a few rubber bands, and the patient's fingers.

CHAPTER IV.

FINGER SQUEEZING FOR EYE TROUBLES.

IF your eyes pain, close them lightly — or leave them open, if you prefer — and squeeze tightly the knuckles of the first (or index) fingers of both hands. Occasionally, if the eyes are set far apart and extend over into the third zone, the second (or middle) finger must be included in this digital embrace. But as a general rule pressure on the upper and lower surfaces, as well as on the sides of the first and second fingers will, within five minutes, relieve the pain of eye strain. Understand, I say "relieve", not "cure". For if the eye strain is the result of a too constant attendance at "movie" shows, and due to the fact that the little eye muscles are expanding and contracting hundreds of times a minute in an attempt to "focus" upon the flickering screen, the only cure for this strain is to "cut out" these entertainments, or else patronize a movie house where the flicker has been "cut out." Of course, if the eye strain is the result of imbalance of the muscles of the eye it will be necessary to properly adjust this faulty

(43)

focus by reinforcing the lens of the eye with a supplementary one made of glass.

But for temporary relief firm pressure over the joints of the first and second fingers, continued for several minutes, will usually give results.

Eye strain and muscle tire are largely under the control of the nervous system. If the nerves are fatigued, the muscles function imperfectly. If the muscles are wearied the nerves sympathize, and make the fact known by raising a wail of distress.

And so it follows that a skeptic is legitimately entitled to say "Yes, you zone therapists cure eye strain by squeezing fingers or toes, but as the condition is primarily a nervous one, you really cure it by suggestion."

This, notwithstanding the fact that frequently the patient has no idea as to what is being attempted, and doesn't, until his pain is relieved, know why any one should want to squeeze his fingers.

Also, I would urgently recommend any believer in the "suggestion" or "mental" response of eye pains to omit pressures over the first and second fingers to try and help this condition by squeezing the thumb and little finger, and see what they accomplish.

However, accepting the extreme position of some of our friends, and admitting that all eye strain is imagination—or an error of the mind—I would ask them to consider the pert, prominent, and resolutely determined stye—which is certainly not imaginary, nor merely suggested. Also inflammatory conditions of the conjunctiva—the membrane of the eye and lids—and that irritating and extremely annoying affliction known as granulated lids.

It might be considered a crucial test of imagination to dissipate and clear up these conditions, yet zone therapy does just this. For sties and such eye conditions as conjunctivitis and granulated lids are completely relieved by pressure exerted upon the joints of the first and second finger of the hand corresponding to the eye involved. In sties the relief is frequently complete in one or two treatments. In other inflammatory conditions of the mucous membranes of the eye it may be necessary to give treatments three times a week for several weeks. Also, a bandage fastened around the index fingers, and soaked with camphor water, frequently relieves itching and congestion of the eyes.

Favorable results are almost routine in these troubles, and usually without employing any other measures. For facilitating treatment, however—unless the results of the exclusive use of zone therapy are desired for experimental reasons,—it might be well to use hot boric acid compresses, or other indicated measures, in addition to the pressures.

To go still farther I might state a fact that every doctor will immediately admit. And this is, that inflammation of the optic nerve—optic neuritis—is most decidedly not imaginary, nor is it, so far as I know, cured by telling the patient that there is nothing the matter with him. As a usual thing, whether treated or not, one afflicted with optic neuritis goes on to complete blindness.

Yet we have cured optic neuritis by making pressures over the first and second fingers, and over the inferior dental nerve—where it enters the lower jaw bone.

One patient I have in mind, who had been treated without benefit by several competent medical men, using conventional and accepted methods, received no other form of treatment— no local applications, no antiseptics. Yet relief followed almost immediately after the pressures were made. The woman was treated twice the first day. That night she slept without taking an opiate—something she had not done before in several weeks.

A complete cure of her condition was brought about within a week, and now, after the expiration of six months, there has been no return of her symptoms.

For the benefit of physician readers I should like to add that in treating eye strain, conjunctivitis, sties, granulated lids, and eye conditions generally, pressures made with a blunt probe, (see E Fig. 11) on the muco-cutaneous margins (where the skin joins the mucous membrane in the nostrils) affects the second division of the opthalmic nerve, and assists materially in bringing about a favorable influence in eye troubles.

I would also emphasize the importance of seeing that the condition of the eye teeth was perfect, as frequently some chronic inflammatory eye trouble may be caused by an infection from the roots of the canine teeth.

In order permanently to cure anything its cause must be removed. And it stands to reason that if a patient persists in poisoning himself with coffee, tobacco, or alcohol; or suffers from an impoverished condition of the blood, or from a brain tumor, lead poisoning, or an injury, or has some constitutional or organic disease or some spinal lesion, which is the basis for his eye trouble, permanent relief will not follow unless these causes are removed or corrected.

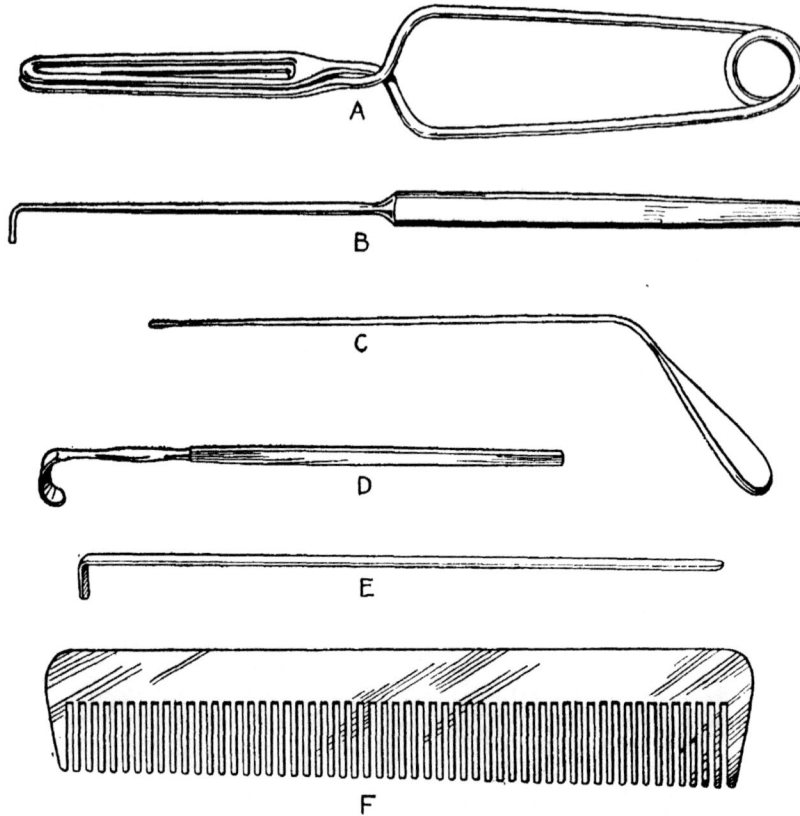

Non-Electrical Applicators Useful in Zone Therapy

A is an ordinary surgical clamp which can be used for clamping the tongue.

B is an ordinary eye-muscle retractor. This can be used for intermittently retracting the posterior pillars of the fauces.

C is a special type of nasal probe used for attacking the posterior wall of the nasopharynx.

D is a regular palpebral retractor which can be used for intermittently retracting the soft palate, especially in the region of the fossa of Rosenmüller.

E is a regular flat applicator bent up at one end. This is useful about the throat and fauces. It can be used as a pressure applicator for the posterior wall of the oropharynx.

F is an ordinary aluminum comb used for attacking the fingers or toes either at the tips or about the joints.

FIG. 11.

But if he has a condition due to an excess of nerve or muscle tension, or if he has trouble produced by faulty circulation from any cause, squeezing his fingers will come nearer to curing him—and more expeditiously and satisfactorily—than any other treatment. If you don't believe it, try it. It costs nothing but a few minutes' intelligent effort.

4

CHAPTER V.

MAKING THE DEAF HEAR.

TOO much knowledge is a dangerous thing. For it keeps one thus afflicted from acquiring more.

Of course it seems outlandish and quite beyond the pale of reason, to ask a man who can minutely describe the semi-circular canals of the ear, or bound the internal labyrinth on the north, south, east and west, to believe that by pressing with a blunt probe behind the wisdom tooth, or at the angle of the jaw on the upper surface, the hearing of the adjacent ear can be materially benefited. Or that a similar result would follow squeezing upon the joints of the ring finger, or the toe corresponding to the ring finger. And this, after every other scientifically accredited method, administered by the world's greatest specialists, had failed. Yet such is the fact. For it is the experience of physicians, familiar with the practice and principles of zone therapy, that nine out of ten cases of otosclerosis (thickening or chronic congestion of the membranes of the ear) can be improved from 25% to 90%.

(50)

And, that ringing in the ears and "ear noises," or catarrhal deafness, can be relieved in an even larger number of cases. If there is any hearing left at all, these methods are almost certain to improve it.

General practitioners, osteopaths and dentists, who do not know so much about the geography of the ear as does the ear specialist, have no hesitation in "trying out" these methods, frequently with astonishing results.

One dentist of my acquaintance, whose knowledge of the ear is merely academic, has cured or materially improved the hearing of more than twenty of his patients. This he did by instructing them to tuck a "wad" of absorbent lint, or a handkerchief, in the space between the last tooth and the angle of the jaw, and "bite down hard" upon this substance for several minutes, repeating this procedure two or three times daily.

Some medical men cause these patients to "work" on the ring finger on the side involved, and do almost as well.

It may better serve our purposes, by way of illustration, were I to cite a few specific cases, and detail their exact manner of treatment. It may then be easier to put the teaching into practical application, following exactly the treatment as outlined.

A lady, the wife of an ear specialist, was recently brought to me for deafness. The doctor, having tried unsuccessfully every accredited method, was constrained to "see what zone therapy would do."

For thirty years this patient had heard nothing with the right ear, and very little with the left. I stimulated, with a stiff, curved cotton-tipped probe (instrument shown in Fig. 6 may be used), the area lying between the last tooth and the angle of the jaw — carefully "covering" all the gum surfaces—sides as well as biting surfaces.

In addition, I hooked an instrument behind the soft palate (see D, Fig. 11), and "stretched" it gently forward. This, I have found, powerfully stimulates the circulation of the "ear zones," and is most helpful—particularly in catarrhal deafness. After two treatments this patient could hear a small tuning fork one-half inch away from the right ear, and one inch from the left. After a few more treatments, her hearing so wonderfully improved that she could hear a whisper with the right ear. This after being "stone deaf" in that ear for thirty years, and after having visited "all the noted aurists in this country and abroad."

A young soprano, member of a leading Hartford church choir, suffered a progressive loss in hearing, which finally became so pronounced as to make it almost impossible for her to "sing on the pitch," or harmonize with either the organ or the other quartette members.

She received treatment similar to that employed on the aurist's wife, supplementing the same by "home treatment." This consisted in "tucking" a wad of surgeon's gauze (it has since been discovered that a solid rubber eraser gives even better results) in the space back of the wisdom tooth, and having her bite forcibly upon it, repeating the procedure several times daily—especially immediately before singing or rehearsing. In a few weeks this girl had completely recovered her hearing, and was able to accept an engagement with a traveling concert company, a position very much more remunerative than the church position she resigned.

I have had to date possibly fifty cases of deafness of one kind or another, almost all of which have been materially helped.

One patient, a minister afflicted with otosclerosis (this supposed thickening of the membranes of the inner ear) for twenty-five years, could barely hear loud talking.

After working for five minutes upon the joints of the third (ring) finger, and to a lesser degree, upon its two neighbors, it was found that the reverend gentleman could hear a whisper twenty feet away.

As proof of this it was whispered to him "Will you kindly close the window above your head?" He rose immediately from his chair, and "obliged."

A New York physician had a relative who had been unsuccessfully treated for deafness in one ear (the right) for the past sixteen years, by the most famous aurists in New York, London, Paris, Berlin, Dresden, Vienna, and other centers of medical learning. X-Ray treatment had at one time made this case at least twenty-five per cent worse. With the left ear this patient could hear a loud voice "close up."

Dr. Reid Kellogg volunteered to "show the Doctor something," using this case for demonstration purposes.

The Doctor, like Barkis, being willin', our friend took his trusty aluminum comb from his pocket and exerted pressure for five minutes with the teeth of the comb on the finger tips of the patient's left hand, (see Fig. 12). He then used a tongue depressor on the hard palate, and on the floor of the mouth, for six or seven minutes more, and then on the tongue for an additional five.

The Doctor then stood ten feet away from his

relative and talked to him in an ordinary tone of
voice. The patient distinctly heard, with the
left ear, every word spoken.

Our pupil then started to work on the other
hand. The patient insisted that this was merely

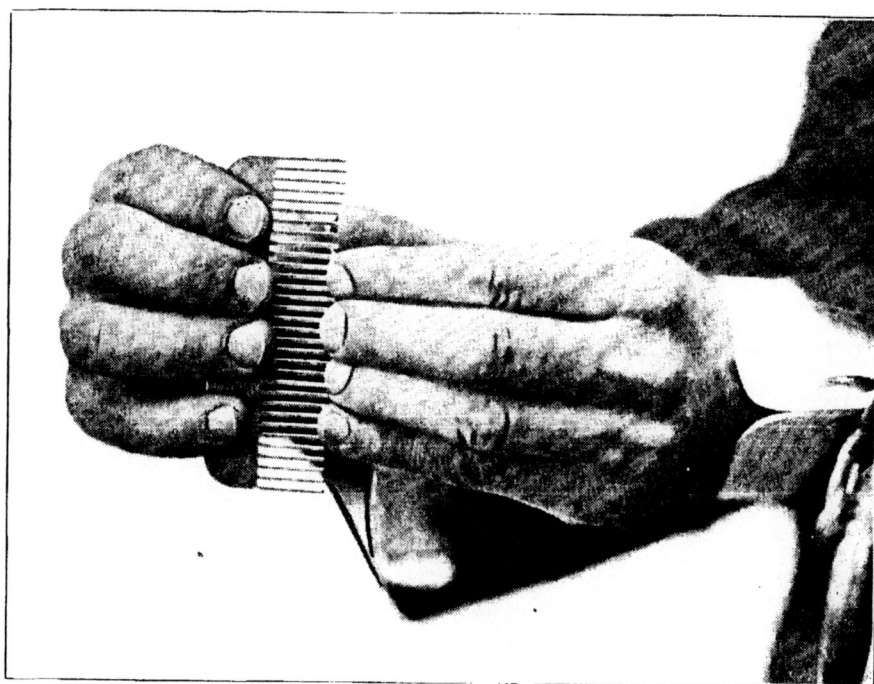

FIG. 12. — This illustrates one method of treating the bones and deep
seated conditions generally. Pressure on the tips of the fingers influences
both anterior and posterior aspects of second, third, fourth and fifth zones.

a waste of time, as the "biggest" ear specialists
in Europe had failed upon this. However, the
attempt was made, and within ten minutes the
patient heard a clock a foot away, a watch held
three inches distant from his ear, and he further

was able to repeat words spoken loudly two feet away. During the experiments with his right ear, the left was tightly plugged with cotton, still further wedged in the canal by the physician's finger. So this was a rather conclusive test.

A lady, aged forty-nine, deaf since she was six years old, came to the office of a specialist who had studied zone therapy. When the physician applied a comb to one hand, she put the other to one side of her lips—the side the doctor was on—and whispered to her friend "Crank." Twenty minutes later, being then able to hear ordinary conversation, she whispered again. This time she said "Wizard." A few days later she asked a friend riding with her in a street car if the bell always rang when the conductor pulled the strap. She was hearing it for the first time in her life.

One lady came to this doctor with her husband. They were both deaf. But the baby in her arms was not deaf—and most decidedly was not dumb either. In less than a fortnight's treatment both parents could hear the baby cry every night, which was a great satisfaction to them— in one way. But they don't know yet whether to laugh or cry about it.

Dr. Thomas Mournighan has given me the details of two remarkable cases, one a veteran of sixty-eight, who, since the Civil War, has been deaf from gun concussion. This man had never heard through the telephone, the perfection and general use of which dates since the war.

After making pressure with a probe (applicator shown in Fig. 6 may be used) on the gum margins near the angle of the jaw this gentleman was able to hear through a 'phone—the first time he had ever experienced this pleasure. That it was a pleasure was evidenced by the fact that the old soldier danced around the office in a perfect transport of glee.

The Doctor's own father, whose condition was similar to that of the other patient, also developed a very material increase in his ability to hear.

It is but fair to say, however, that the patient's "home treatments" must be persistent in order to maintain this improvement. If these treatments are discontinued for any appreciable length of time the condition seems to relapse. We are not yet prepared to say why this should be so.

I would emphasize also that, in ear trouble, the condition of wisdom teeth be carefully looked after. For, I am convinced, many cases of loss of hearing, or middle ear trouble, have their origin in some pathological condition of these teeth.

It may be of interest here to note also that one of the most effective ear-ache cures we possess is a spring clothespin fastened for five minutes or thereabouts on the tip of the ring finger. (See Fig. 13.) Any manipulation over this zone is effective, but hollowed-out spring clothespins and rubber bands have been particularly so.

To illustrate: During a recent medical convention in the West one of the physicians attending complained of a severe ear-ache. A physician present, well versed in zone therapy, requested permission to examine the ear-ache doctor's fingers, alleging that by pressing intermittently on the finger nails, he could estimate the degree of blood pressure, and perhaps suggest a course of treatment which might permanently cure the ear trouble—if not caused by an abscess.

The doctor extended the hand on the side of the afflicted ear.

The zone therapy man squeezed the tip of the fourth finger, raised the finger nail, and let it settle back a dozen or more times, "to see how the circulation reacted," as he said. After three or

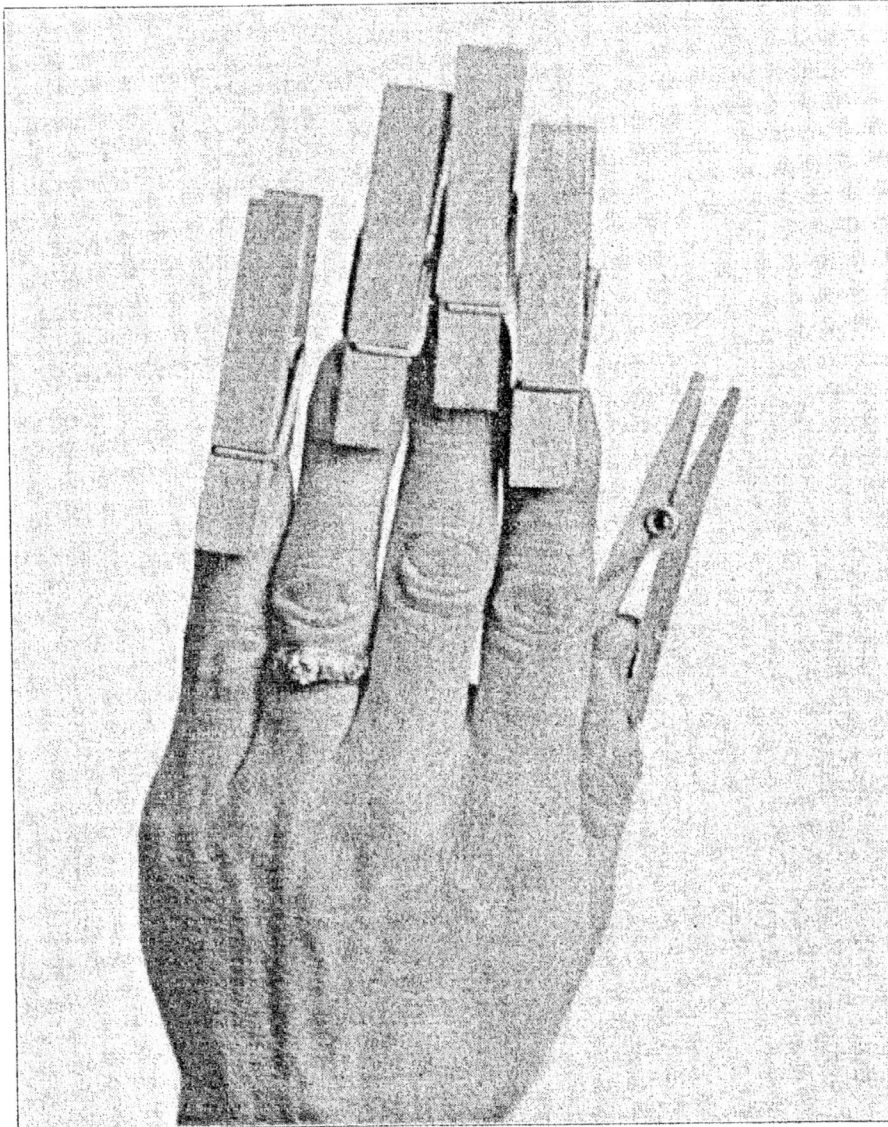

FIG. 13. — Showing method of applying hollowed out spring clothes pins for the relief of pain and to desensitize the teeth for dental operations.

four minutes he said "By the way, Doctor, which ear did you say is giving you the trouble?"

The Doctor looked up in blank amazement, felt his ears, shook his head, and said, "You don't mean to say that that darned foolishness cured my ear-ache, do you?"

It does seem silly, and yet it "works." And anything that works is beneficent and helpful, and deserves encouragement. For deafness and ear troubles are common, and seem to be becoming more so.

CHAPTER 6.

PAINLESS CHILDBIRTH.

ANY method, no matter how improbable-seeming it may be, calculated to render labor or operations upon women less of an ordeal, is worthy of consideration by physicians, midwives, and the laity. Therefore there may be something well worth "trying out" in the "pressure" method of inducing relief from pain.

A number of physicians have reported results that, if confirmed by further experiences, warrant us in believing that zone pressure promises to be a boon to womankind.

To those who have had experience with pressure analgesia in dentistry, and in the relief of rheumatism, lumbago, neuralgia, and other painful affections, mitigating—or even entirely relieving—the pains of childbirth seem quite within the bounds of possibility. In any event, it will not be difficult to put it to a broad conclusive test. And it is absolutely harmless, there is no danger to mother or child in its employment, and no indication that it might be responsible for a "blue baby." For in almost every case in which it has

(61)

been tried, labor has been accelerated six hours or more—instead of retarded.

The methods are so simple that they can be utilized by any one—even by women who may, in their hour of labor, chance to be remote from medical attention. Two combs (broad aluminum combs about four inches in length have been found to be the best) to clench the fingers and thumbs over (see Fig. 14), and some sharp or edged surface to press the soles of the feet against (see Fig. 15), are all the instruments that are required, altho a clamp has now been devised (see Fig. 16) which can be fastened on the hands to include both surfaces and all zones. It is applied when contractions begin, and is kept in position intermittently until delivery is completed. Rubber bands, bound around the great and "index" toes, also afford a gratifying help.

To relieve the after-pains and facilitate the expulsion of the afterbirth, it has been found that "stimulating" strokes, with the teeth of the aluminum comb, or the "bristles" of a wire hair brush, are most effective. It may require that these strokes be given from ten minutes to one-half hour. But they assist wonderfully in contracting the uterus.

Dr. R. T. H. Nesbitt, of Waukegan, Ill., is one of a number of physicians who have had

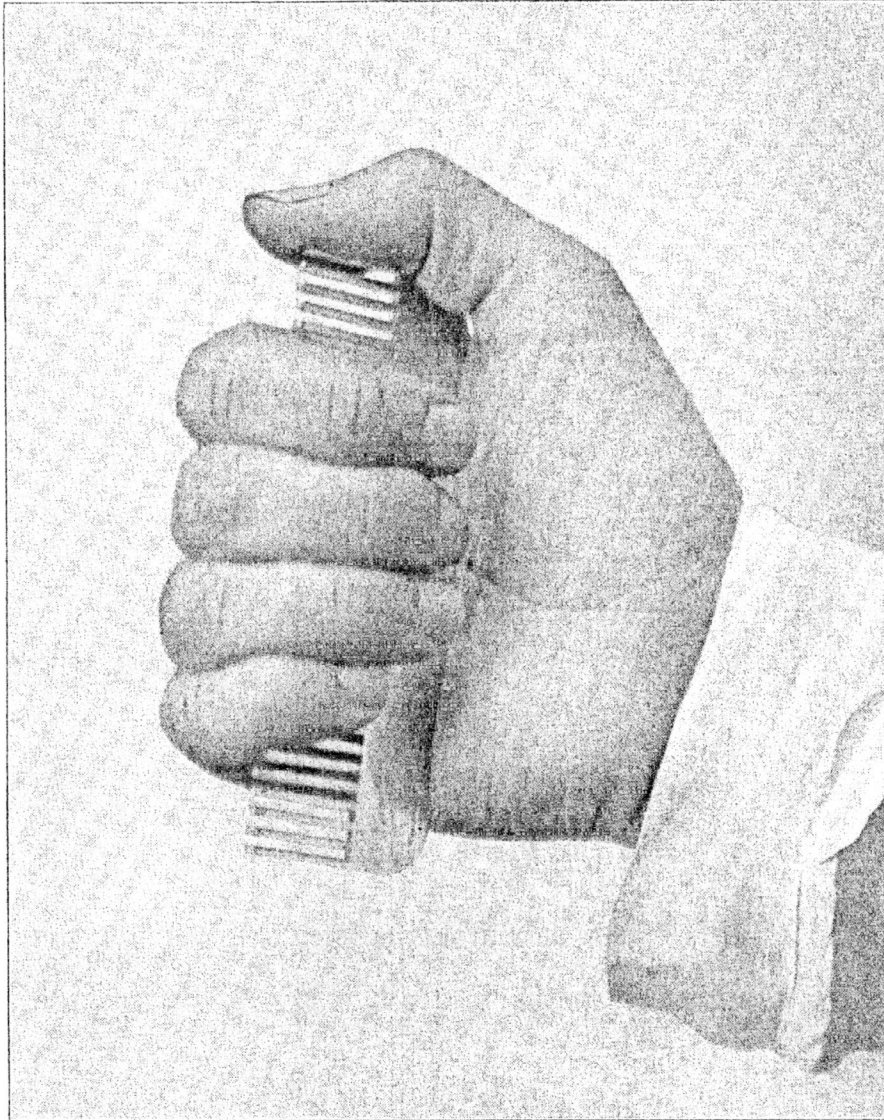

FIG. 14. — This shows method of treating lumbago and pains in the back of the body, affecting all the zones.

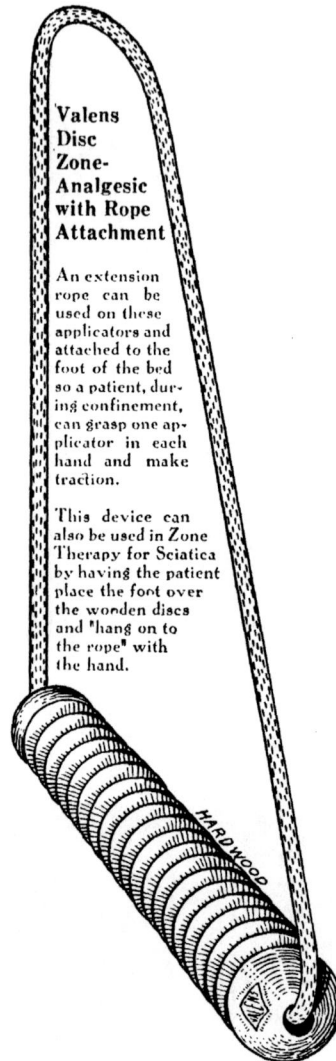

Valens
Disc
Zone-
Analgesic
with Rope
Attachment

An extension
rope can be
used on these
applicators and
attached to the
foot of the bed
so a patient, dur-
ing confinement,
can grasp one ap-
plicator in each
hand and make
traction.

This device can
also be used in Zone
Therapy for Sciatica
by having the patient
place the foot over
the wooden discs
and "hang on to
the rope" with
the hand.

HARDWOOD

FIG. 15.

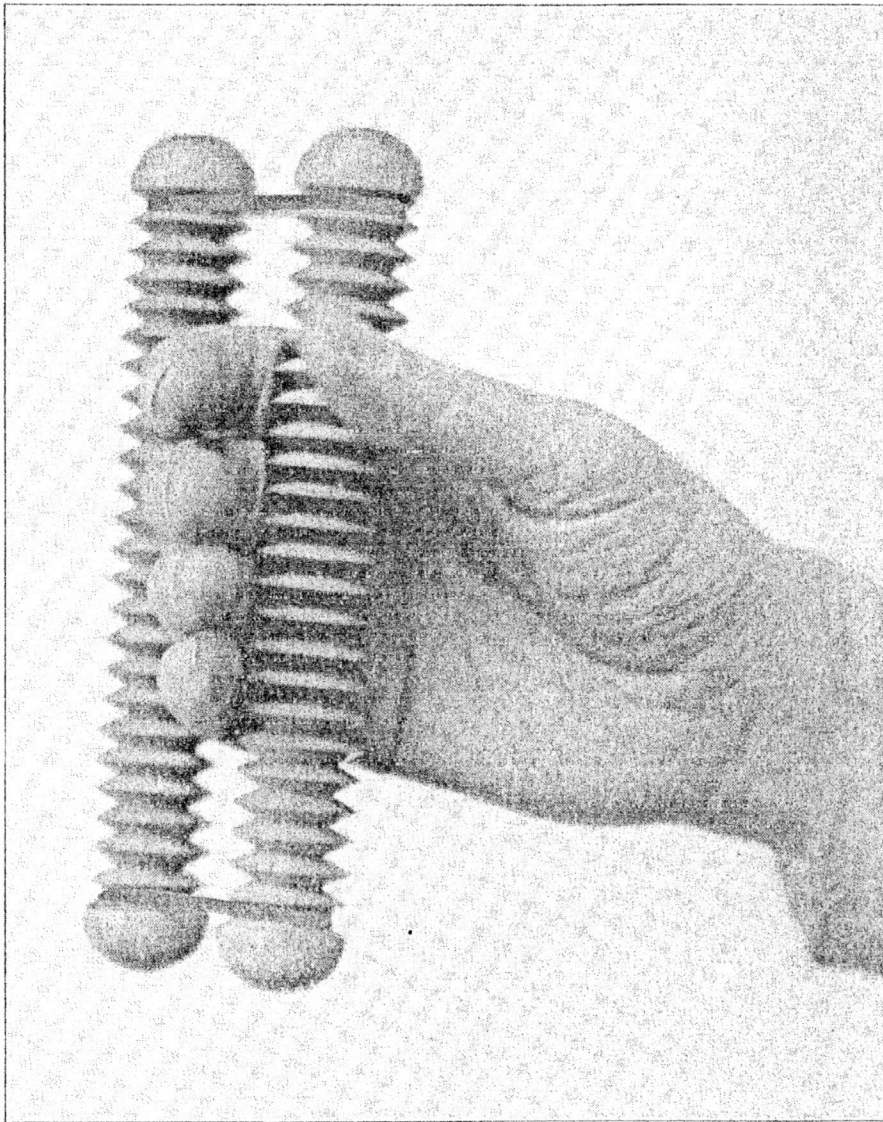

FIG. 16. — This is the hand clamp used with such extraordinary success in relieving the pains of childbirth.

practical experience with pressure analgesia in childbirth.   He sends this very interesting report:

"During the past week I have been attending the lectures of Dr. George Starr White.   In this most interesting and helpful series, Dr. White explained and exemplified biodynamic diagnosis by means of the magnetic meridian (a remarkable discovery of Dr. White, which enables one to diagnose diseases otherwise undiagnosible.   This by means of changes in the "tension" of organs—which occurs when a properly grounded patient is turned from North or South to East or West).   Dr. White also demonstrated zone therapy.   He asked if any of the doctors present expected a confinement case soon.   If so, he wished to give them some suggestions in zone anesthesia in connection with delivery.

"As I was expecting a 'call' every hour I told Dr. White, and he gave me some special points concerning this work.   Last night I was called to attend what I expected would be my last case in confinement, as I have been doing this work so many years that I intended to retire.   From my last night's experience I feel as if I should like to start the practice of medicine all over again.

"The woman I delivered was a primipara

(one who had never had a child before, and who therefore, because of the rigidity of the bones and tissues, has a more difficult labor), small in stature.

"When severe contractions began, and the mother was beginning to be very nervous and complained of pain, at which time I generally administer chloroform, I began pressing on the soles of the feet with the edge of a big file, as I could find nothing else. I pressed on the top of the foot with the thumbs of both hands at the metatarsal-phalangeal joint, (where the toes join the foot). I exerted this pressure over each foot for about three minutes at a time. The mother told me that the pressure on the feet gave her no pain whatsoever.

"As she did not have any uterine pain, I was afraid there was no advancement. To my great surprise, when I examined her about ten or fifteen minutes later, I found the head within two inches of the outlet. I then waited about fifteen minutes, and on examination found the head at the vulva. I then pressed again for about one or two minutes on each foot, the edge of the file being on the sole of the foot, and my thumbs over the tarsal-metatarsal joints as before. In this way I exerted pressure on the sole of the foot with the file, and pressure on the dorsum of the foot with my thumbs, doing each foot separately. The last pressure lasted about one and a half minutes to each foot. Within five or ten minutes the head was appearing, and I held it back to preserve the perineum (the tissue joining the vagina and the rectum). It made steady progress, the head and shoulders coming out in a normal manner. Within three minutes the child—which "weighed in" at 9 1/2 pounds—was born, crying lustily. The mother told me she did not experience any pain whatever, and could not believe the child was born. She laughed and said, 'This is not so bad.'

"Another point that is very remarkable is that after the child was born, the woman did not experience the fatigue that is generally felt, and the child was more active than usual. I account for this on the principle that pain inhibits (prevents) progress of the birth, and tires the child. But as the pain was inhibited, the progress was more steady, and thus fatigue to both mother and child was avoided."

A Massachusetts doctor supplements this case with several others—equally ridiculous or revolutionary—depending upon our viewpoint. To insure brevity and accuracy I quote the Doctor's own words.

"Case 1. Multipara (a woman who has had

previous confinements)—mother of four. Shortest previous labor eight hours. Had had a laceration of cervix (neck of the womb) with her first child. Also one forceps delivery.

"When labor commenced she was given two aluminum combs to hold (as shown in Fig. 14), and instructed to make strong pressure upon them, with a view of inhibiting pains, particularly in the first, second and third zones. These combs were four inches in length and slightly roughened on the ends, so that the lateral (or side) surfaces of the thumbs could more effectively be stimulated.

"Was called at four a. m., arrived at 5:05, and the babe had just been born. The patient reported that she had been in bed for only 15 minutes. There had been only one severe pain. This was when the head delivered.

"There was no exhaustion following, as with her previous labors, and she said laughingly, 'I believe I'll be able to get up this afternoon, Doctor.'

"The afterbirth delivery seemed to be stimulated, and the pains controlled by stroking the backs of the hands with the teeth of the combs. She became relaxed and drowsy from this stroking, and finally fell asleep and slept almost through the night—perfectly free from pain.

"Case 2. Primipara, thirty-seven years old.
This woman had a badly retroflexed uterus (a
womb which is tilted back), which seemed to re-
tard the advancement of labor, for she required
five hours for delivery.

"She also used the comb pressures, and, in addition, was provided with a rough-edged shal-
low box, upon which she pressed firmly with the
soles of her feet.

"Four hours after delivery she had sharp
afterbirth pains, which were controlled by the
stroking method before described. This seemed
to give complete and satisfactory relaxation.

"There were three other cases, all of which
responded equally well to treatment by zone
analgesia.

"It should be added that, while the pain was
inhibited, there seemed to be no diminution in
the strength of the uterine contractions."

Dr. Thomas Mournighan, of Providence, R.
I., has been, for more than two years, one of the
staunchest advocates of my methods. He has
had phenomenally successful experiences in
goiter, deafness, female irregularities, and in the
relief of pain and cure of conditions in the general practice of medicine.

Dr. Mournighan has also had almost uniformly successful results with zone analgesia in childbirth. I quote from a few of his cases.

"Case 1. Primipara, nineteen years of age. Suffered from furious attacks of vomiting at the beginning of her pregnancy. Her family physician wanted to abort her, fearing for her life, unless the attacks were checked.

"She finally came under my care. I instructed her to bite her tongue as hard as she could, about one-third the distance from the tip—thus, as you see, 'attacking' the entire zone connection. This procedure controlled the vomiting almost immediately, and instead of becoming accustomed to it, thereby losing its beneficial effect, she became, if anything, even more susceptible to its influence.

"When she came to term I placed a rough-edged box in the bed, for her to press the soles of her feet on. I also provided her with a sheet, tied to the bed post, which she gripped and pulled upon during pains. This, I feel certain, helps pain relief by zone analgesia—as well as by assisting in the mechanics of labor. She made traction upon the sheets and pressed her feet on the box as the condition seemed to require, and, as she expressed it, 'got great comfort from it.'

"When the second stage of labor came on—

that stage where I generally resort to chloroform
—I made strong pressure over the feet, sinking
my thumbs well in over the articulation of the
toe and foot joint. She was delivered in less
than five hours. The afterbirth came away without the slightest pain. I was peculiarly struck
by the almost complete absence of labor exhaustion."

"Case 2. Mother aged forty, ninth child. She
had had 'the devil's own time' with the last three
or four, the attendant having been compelled to
use forceps in these births. With her last child
she had had a bad laceration of the cervix,
which, however, had been skillfully repaired.

"I gave her two aluminum combs, the edges
of which I had nicked with a file, so as to
roughen them for the thumb to press over.
There being no box handy I covered a coal
shovel with a towel, and, when the pains became severe, let her press the soles of her feet
against the sharp edge of this.

"Within 3 hours she was delivered—without
forceps this time—of a 10½ pound boy—as clean
a delivery as I ever saw.

"I know it seems crazy, but any method that
will, practically without pain, stimulate women
who were formerly in labor for from twelve to
fifteen hours to complete delivery—in many in-

stances within three hours— is a good method. I shall continue its use, no matter how foolish it may appear."

Another physician, who has had a large and successful experience with zone therapy, writes:

"In obstetrics I have almost completely discarded chloroform at the close of the second stage, where I used to almost always use it. In the first stage, zone therapy relieves the nagging pains without retarding, but rather promoting dilatation. In the second stage delivery is hastened. Women seem so quiet and easy one would think 'there was nothing doing,' until on examination, you are surprised to see what has been accomplished. For this work I use a serrated strip of aluminum 1/16 in. thick, imbedded in a piece of wood of convenient size, or else I use a seven inch aluminum comb, pressing the teeth against the inner part of the sole of the foot, or near the ball, alternating from one foot to the other. When I have an assistant both feet are manipulated at a time, and that aids very materially. I exert as much pressure as the patient can bear without pain. When I have an assistant well trained I am going to try zone therapy for instrumental delivery."

In connection with the subject of confinement and operations upon women this report from

Dr. G. Murray Edwards, of Denver, Colorado, is of peculiar interest:

"Mrs. McK., age 35; pregnant four and a half months; multipara. Placenta praevia (a grave condition, in which the afterbirth precedes the child in delivery), aborted Dec. 5, 1915, curettement (scraping out of the uterus), Dec. 7, 1915. Temperature 99, pulse 80. This case occurring during Dr. White's lecture course in Denver, when Dr. Fitzgerald's pressure method of analgesia was being discussed, I decided to try it out for the first time on this patient. She being a very nervous woman, I felt a little reluctant in the experiment. I did not tell her, however, I was going to use a new method, but quietly placed three elastics, an eighth of an inch wide, on each foot, one around the large toe at the first joint, and one around the others similarly in pairs.

"After fifteen minutes, preparing my instruments in the meantime, I told her we were ready, and while we did not intend to use chloroform, instructed her carefully to tell me immediately if she felt any pain whatsoever. The curettement was conducted in every detail as though she were under general anesthesia, and as I questioned her frequently as to pain, she always came back with a smile and a negative reply.

"We removed fully a teacupful of placental tissue in about ten minutes, while the patient passed the time joking, and when finished assured me she felt much better than when we started, as she was nervous looking forward to the anesthetic. This I consider a typical case, and have no misgivings as to its working generally."

In similar strain scores of letters tell of the successes attending the employment of this method in labor, and in operations upon women.

Now, I do not contend that a few score, or a few hundred swallows make a summer, but their presence undoubtedly indicates that summer may be well on the way.

All this may sound foolish in the extreme. Yet there are many other things equally foolish in the practice of medicine. And if zone analgesia will do what we claim for it, it may well be taken gently by the hand, lifted out of the foolish class, and placed among the ultra-sensible procedures—where, by right, it belongs.

CHAPTER 7.

ZONE THERAPY FOR WOMEN.

IN the eternal fitness of things there would be something radically wrong if zone therapy did not offer some especial and particular help to women. It is a satisfaction to state that the eternal fitness of things is right, as usual. For zone therapy is as unique in this connection as in most of its other applications.

Many of the things it does are positively startling. And yet they become commonplace, after one has been in the work for a time. One of the most striking cases that has yet come to my attention came in the form of a letter of thanks from a mother of a young girl. I never saw either. The mother, however, wrote me that her daughter, who had not menstruated in ten months, was, some time ago, instructed by a patient of mine to take the broad handle of a tablespoon and make strong pressure upon the tongue (a tongue depressor shown in Fig. 17 would be more appropriate), as far back as she could stand it without gagging.

She did so, and within five minutes was menstruating profusely, yet without the slightest pain or discomfort. In the several months which had since intervened, she "came around" regularly every twenty-eight days. The mother who feared that her daughter was going into a decline, could not refrain from writing me a

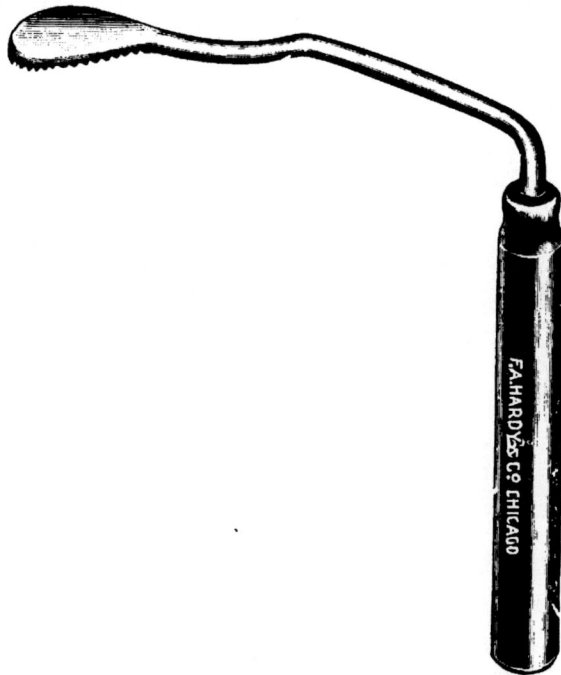

Fig. 17. Tongue-pressor Electrode. May be used with or without electricity.

most heartfull letter of appreciation for what my patient, through my instruction, had been able to do for her daughter. I call this good preventive medicine.

Painful menstruation (dysmenorrhoea), also yields like magic to the potent pressure of a probe applied to the posterior (back) wall of the pharynx. But the tongue pressures are, in the majority of cases, quite as effective. For pain in the back or thighs, preceding or during menstruation, pressure with the tip of the index finger on the posterior wall of the pharynx on the median line and to the right and left of same, will almost uniformly give relief.

A broad, rough-surfaced tongue depressor (see Fig. 17) is best for the purpose. But if this is not available, the handle of a large spoon or the handle of a tooth brush may be used.

This should be applied to the tongue three-quarters of the way back and on the median line. The patient's head should be held rigid, and the lower jaw supported, to the end that stronger pressure can be made. It is well to have the physician or some male member of the family officiate in this, as the patient may not be inclined to use the requisite amount of force.

The pressure should be held firmly for two minutes. Then it should be relaxed and the point of focus changed slightly. Or the instrument may be turned or rotated from side to side, at one minute intervals.

Many patients who are obliged to go to bed for two or three days each month, after a course of this treatment, are completely relieved of all distress. Indeed, some of these hardly knew they were "coming sick."

It might be added that pressure exerted on the thumb, first and second fingers of both hands helps materially in this work. And one of the most comforting factors in the practice is that patients are usually quite as well the next morning as they are even directly after the most successful treatment.

Occasionally the use of the metal comb on the back of the hand, "combing" thoroly the region of the thumb, first and second fingers as far as to the wrists—has given best results. But the tongue pressures are most uniformly successful.

While I have seldom heard of a miscarriage being induced by these pressures, yet I believe a note of warning should be sounded, cautioning against the use of the tongue pressures, particularly during the early months of pregnancy.

For it is quite conceivable that abortion might follow drastic tongue treatment. It would be far better during these months to depend upon the finger pressures or the comb for treatment of these zones.

Also, if there is a too-profuse and too-frequent menstruation, severe tongue pressures should be avoided. In these conditions gentle stroking on the backs of the hands with a wire hair brush or the teeth of the metal comb has given best results. And this same procedure may be confidently resorted to to prevent threatened abortion.

While not confined to women, yet women are by far more generally afflicted with constipation and hemorrhoids than are men. Their sedentary habits, tight lacing, and repugnance to water drinking make them peculiarly susceptible to the costive habit—which in turn, through engorgement of the hemorrhoidal veins, causes piles.

I mention these subjects here because the treatment for constipation and hemorrhoids is identical with that given for painful or suppressed menstruation.

The results in constipation are, in some instances, absolutely astonishing. I know of one woman, constipated for fifteen years, who never knew what it meant to have a natural movement of the bowels. She grasped the chair seat with the tips of her fingers and thumbs, putting all her strength into this grip — so as partly to desensitize the pain of tongue pressure, and thereby be able to stand a more drastic treatment. Then the tongue was firmly pressed for nine minutes in the manner before described.

Her bowels moved within fifteen minutes

afterwards, and for a year or longer she has never had to take another cathartic. Another case was cleared up two years ago, and has had no return of the former trouble.

These, however, are the extraordinary and exceptional cases. For routine treatment it may be well to use the pressures for a considerable period of time, so that their stimulating effect may tend to create a "habit" in the peristaltic muscles of the bowel. For the cure cannot be considered complete until this "habit" is firmly established.

The pain, bleeding and swelling of piles is also helped by these same procedures.

The point to be most emphatically dwelt upon in connection with the treatment of these conditions is that "absent treatment," or lick-and-a-promise namby-pambyism, isn't of any avail. The pressures must be made by some one who has more sympathy with the patient's ultimate good than he has for her present temporary discomfort, and who will administer a good honest treatment—preferably while the patient does all she can—by tightly clasping the hands on the interlocked fingers, or by grasping the chair or a table with the finger tips—to reduce the sensitivity of the zones operated upon.

6

If zone therapy is used in this manner, the results will amaze and delight. For no method yet evolved for the treatment of these disorders even remotely approximates zone therapy in point of efficacy.

CHAPTER 8.

RELAXING NERVOUS TENSION.

PERHAPS you may not do it. You have such splendid control over yourself. But you know many people who, when angry, or when suffering great physical pain, sink their teeth into their lip. Sometimes they bite hard enough to start the blood. Others clinch their teeth and hands, and double their toes up in their shoes. Why do you suppose they do this? They do these, and many other natural and apparently inevitable things, because they are instinctive and scientific, and because Nature knows her business. We have done and shall continue to do them involuntarily and automatically, because they relieve pain and nerve tension, because they produce a form of analgesia, or pain-deadening, similar to that which follows the injection of water or some anesthetic solution into a sensory nerve. If you stop and think for a moment many examples of this inhibition—as it is called—will recur.

One of the most interesting, from our standpoint, was that of a young school teacher, subject to cataleptic fits, who, when she felt one of her fits coming on, stepped on her right toes with all the weight she could throw on the left foot, at the same time grasping the right wrist firmly. Often those near—if notified in time—would produce the pressures for her. In this way the young woman managed to break up or prevent all except severe and sudden attacks.

It was subsequently found that this patient had a chronic irritation in the right ovary, and also a strained condition of the muscles of accommodation in the right eye. When these conditions were cleared up by proper remedial measures and correction, the cataleptic attacks ceased.

The fact of relief having followed in many instances her "inhibiting" the right-sided zones indicated the possible source of trouble. And by painstakingly examining the organs in these zones the cause of her condition was located and finally overcome.

So, as a means of diagnosis zone therapy has an immense value. Its curative effects, however, are most valuable and significant. Many of the gravest nerve conditions — conditions which failed to respond to the most skilled medical treatment obtainable anywhere—have been completely and permanently cured by the application of the proper pressures—properly made.

I recall a very grave case of neurosis — a writer's cramp—accompanying a neurasthenic condition. This lady—unusually alert and intelligent—was a physical and nervous wreck. Sleepless, harassed by "nerves" in their most aggravated form, she was unable to hold a pen, or to write more than a few minutes at a time, until, on account of the pain and twitching of the arm, wrist, and fingers, she was forced to desist. She could no more have picked up and threaded a needle—let alone have sewed with it—than she could have operated an aeroplane. She was also nearly deaf from a middle ear trouble.

Several months' treatment, using the aluminum comb across the front and back of the hands and on the finger tips, and daily employment of the tongue depressor for four or five minutes, brought about a complete change in the patient's condition.

It relaxed the terrible nervous tension—which was particularly marked along the course of the spine—enabling her to sleep at night, and awake thoroly rested and refreshed in the morning. The writer's cramp was also completely cleared up. A number of other conditions were also corrected, and the hearing was improved quite 50%.

This lady has since resumed her occupation as a private secretary—a position she was forced by

ill health to relinquish more than two years ago—
and now writes for hours at a stretch, without
any return of the cramp in the hand and arm.

And, most convincing of all, she can now not
only pick up, thread, and hold a needle—something she had not been able to do for years—
but she can sew steadily for two or three hours,
and feel no disagreeable effects from this fem-
inine debauch.

A peculiarly satisfactory characteristic in all
these cases is that the improvement is even more
apparent the "morning after" than it is immediately after the treatment.

Another case of neuritis in the arm and
shoulder (brachial neuritis) for more than six
years had been unable to raise his arm higher
than the shoulder. For the two months previous
to treatment he had been obliged to carry it in a
sling. The slightest movement of the arm brought
about a paroxysm of agonizing pain.

A number of hollowed-out spring clothespins
were clamped on the fingers of the affected arm
(see Fig. 13), and left there for twelve minutes.
At the expiration of this time the clamps were
removed.

The patient gingerly took his arm from its support, and after a minute or two spent in experimenting with it, moved it freely up behind his

head and swung it behind his back in a sweeping motion.

It was subsequently found that this man also had an osteopathic lesion, which was reduced by Dr. Reid Kellogg, and after a few weeks' "home treatment."—consisting of five minute applications of moderately tight rubber bands around the ends of the fingers—he reported himself as well—and has remained so for more than ten months.

For sciatic neuritis it is found that deep pressures with the teeth of an aluminum or steel comb made upon the toes are much more effective than when made upon the fingers. When pain is most severe on the back of the leg pressures should be made upon the ball (sole) of the foot. (See Fig. 18.) When the front of the leg pains also, the top of the foot should also be pressed.

While we are on the subject of sciatica, I might emphasize the importance of a careful examination of the condition of the wisdom teeth. For very frequently we have found this to be the origin of the sciatic nerve trouble.

Another interesting case, successfully treated with clothespins, was that of a young man suffering from hand tremors, insomnia, and nervous exhaustion.

He had his finger tips clamped daily for a

week. Then three times more, at intervals of three days. After the eighth treatment he had no further trouble with tremor, slept like a baby, and was apparently relieved of all nervous symptoms.

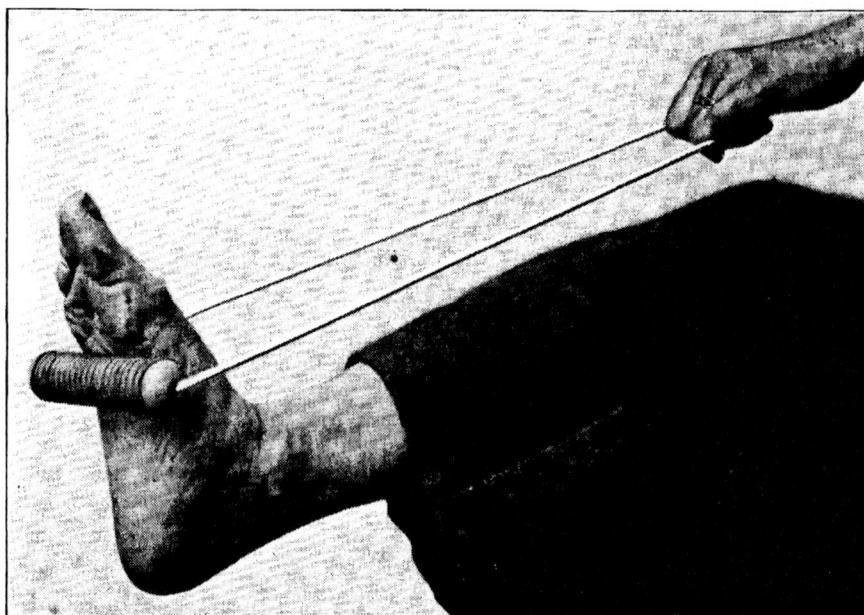

FIG. 18. — Showing a method of treating rheumatism or sciatica by treating all five zones on the back of the leg and body.

We have found it helpful, if the patient has a good set of teeth, to have him clinch the teeth, and also the hands, for several minutes at a time, three or four times daily. This produces an exaggerated degree of relaxation, which is most helpful in overcoming nervous conditions.

Most of our patients are also instructed to "yawn prodigiously," and stretch. This stimulates a healthy action of the sympathetic nerves in all the zones, and cannot fail but be most beneficial. Sometimes the insomnia of neurasthenia may be effectively overcome by tightly clasping the hands — interlocking the fingers as shown in Fig. 19, or pressing the finger tips firmly together, and holding this position for ten or fifteen minutes — unless sleep should come before this and relax the clasp.

Also, the clinching or wriggling of the toes is of benefit to a neurasthenic. In fact, I am convinced that the method of relieving fatigue in marching troops, discovered by Drs. DeFleury and Jacques — of the French army, is largely an application of the principles of zone therapy.

The French surgeon's idea is temporarily to expel the blood from the legs by raising them. The soldiers remove their shoes and lie prone on the ground, close to a tree or wall, with heads slightly elevated. They then raise their legs against the wall, stretching upwards as far as limb limitations permit.

In this attitude the toes and ankles are worked or "wriggled" briskly. Then the knees are flexed and extended a half dozen times or more.

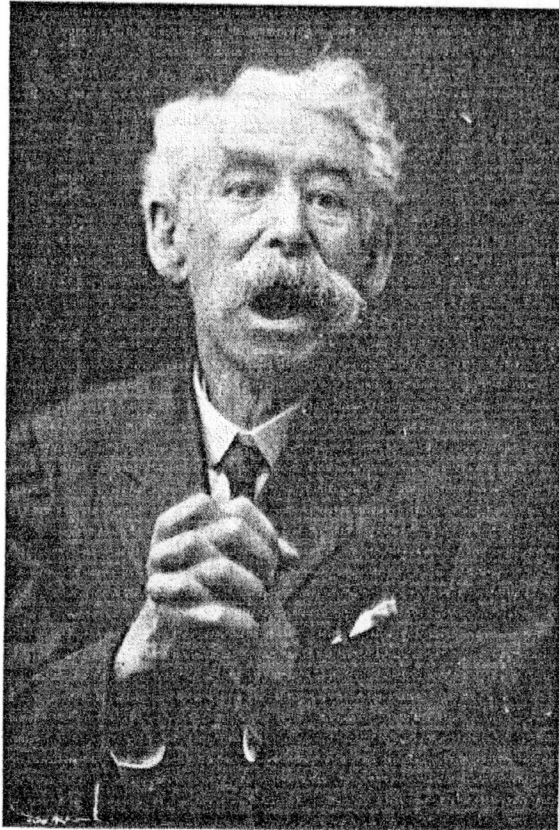

FIG. 19. — Patient seventy-two years of age with carcinoma of left side of tongue, jaw, and pharynx. Two days before this picture was taken the patient was unable to open his mouth. The folded hands and open mouth indicate not only relaxation of the jaws, but the method in which it was brought about. Dr. J. W. Hogan painlessly extracted eighteen teeth for this patient under pressure anesthesia.

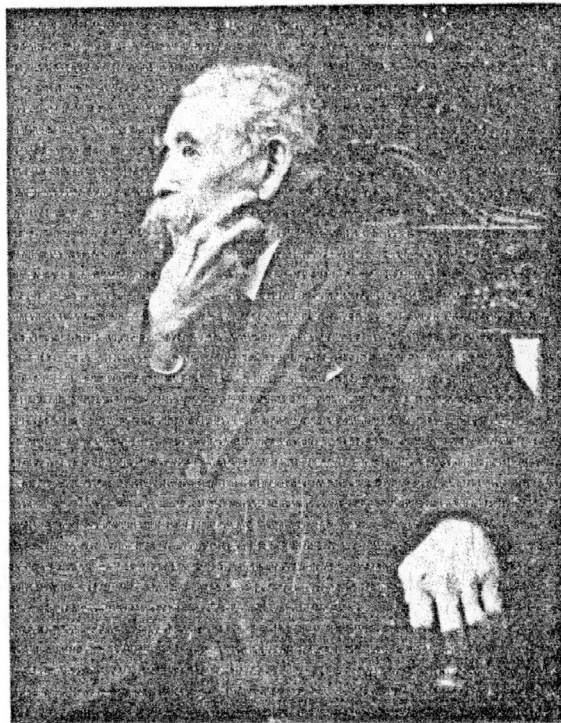

FIG. 20. — Patient with right hand in this picture is indicating with index and middle finger the location of his pain, and how he is overcoming it thru pressure on the arm of the chair with the tips of the thumb and fingers of the left hand. We seldom are obliged to resort to drugs for pain, even in malignancy.

A body of men, apparently in the last stages of exhaustion, recuperate their energies with from five to fifteen minutes' exercise of this kind.

It can readily be seen how, by these exercises, all the zones in the body would be stimulated to a normal condition. And the fact that the exercises practiced are successful on a wholesale scale proves the principle sound.

One of the most important things Americans have to learn is how to relax. Anything that will teach them to do this should prove a boon.

Therefore I feel certain that, before many years, the principles and practices of zone therapy will be as familiar and universally applied as are now the principles of domestic hygiene or the practice of sterilizing baby bottles. And then zone therapy will add to the depth and breadth, as well as to the length of human life.

CHAPTER IX.

CURING LUMBAGO WITH A COMB.

THERE is a solid and substantial satisfaction in having lumbago. For we know, without being told, that we have it, and we don't have to work our imagination overtime providing it with symptoms.

Also, lumbago offers less encouragement to mental or psychological healing than most anything ordinary we could gather up — except a broken leg, a crop of boils, or an abscessed tooth. And the same thing applies to its sisters-in-laws, rheumatism and sciatica.

Therefore, anything that cures lumbago, rheumatism, sciatica, or similar afflictions, must be able to "deliver the goods."

On this basis zone therapy must be considered one of our most valuable methods for treating these obstinate conditions. Naturally it is not always successful. Neither are the salicylates, hot mud baths, porous plasters, nor having teeth pulled. And this is no more an apology for zone therapy than it is for medicine.

Lumbago, as a rule, responds very quickly and

(93)

kindly to zone therapy. Cases which come to the office "all doubled up" are straightened out — frequently in one treatment — and wend their homeward way rejoicing.

The weapon which has given us best results in attacking lumbago and kindred affections is a common, dull-pointed aluminum comb, such as may be procured in most bird stores for dog-combing purposes. The teeth of this are pressed firmly on the palms of the hands and on the palmar surface of the thumb, first, second and third fingers. In order to get the best results the pressures should be continued for from ten to twenty minutes. Occasionally it may be necessary to work also on the "web" between the thumb and first finger, and also between the first and second finger.

Some zone therapy enthusiasts prefer to begin operations on the tips of the thumb, first, second and third fingers — gradually working up the palms of the hands and spending five minutes — for good measure — on the wrists.

Remember always that the palmar surfaces of the hands and fingers are to be attacked for pains anywhere on the back, and the top or (back) surfaces of the hands and fingers for any trouble on the front of the body, arms or legs. This may seem rather confusing at first, but a little thought will make clear why, what are commonly known as the back of the hands are really the front or top, and correspond with the front or top of the feet. The palms of the hands correspond with the soles of the feet.

It is also interesting to note that frequently there are found areas which are extra sensitive to the pressures of the comb.

These areas correspond to the most painful zones in other sections of the body. For instance, if firm pressure on palmar surfaces of right hand elicits more pain through the third zone in the hand, if the patient has already complained of pain in his back, such pain will usually be found in the third zone, and this holds good where pain is concerned throughout the body.

If these sensitive areas are found, by commencing gently and gradually increasing the force of the pressure, toleration can be established. In developing this toleration, the lumbag is usually relieved.

Some perfectly amazing results have been reported from the comb method of treatment, particularly in lumbago. One case, a minister who, for weeks, had been unable even to turn in bed without assistance, was, after a twenty-minute treatment, able to arise and walk unaided. He was entirely relieved of pain and discomfort within a few hours, and the next day was "'up and around." Relief almost always follows the first treatment, apparently irrespective as to the cause of the lumbago. I recall a recent case which had persisted for more than three months. This gentleman had taken practically every form of treatment that could be recommended by the most able specialists, had even been to Hot Springs, without any except transient benefit. He was bent almost double, and for many weeks had not been able to stand erect. This patient was given two aluminum combs and told to squeeze them for ten or fifteen minutes, while waiting in the ante-room. After being brought into the office, his hands were thoroly "combed" by pressure, from finger tip to wrist.

He straightened out completely after this first treatment, and expressed himself as entirely relieved from pain. He received a similar treatment the following day — after which he went his way rejoicing.

These results are practically uniform. I know of many scores of patients thus cured with a comb.

Sometimes equally good results follow from fastening hollowed-out spring clothespins on the tips of the fingers (Fig. 13), corresponding to the zones in which the lumbago holds forth. Or even from binding heavy bands around these fingers (Fig. 5) — leaving these in position five or ten minutes at a time — unless the finger becomes badly discolored sooner, in which case the pressure must be temporarily removed.

One zone therapy enthusiast, who claims that "Treat It By Zone Therapy" should be hung in every doctor's office, while on a pilgrimage to a Shriners' Convention, noticed that the conductor of the train walked "all doubled up" and seemed to be suffering great pain. It developed that the railroad man had a "misery in his back," had given up work, and had been in a sanitarium for three weeks — without obtaining much relief — and also that for the three days prior to his resuming work, he had not been able to "straighten up," nor make any sudden move, without suffering excruciatingly.

He was invited to come into the smoking compartment for a few minutes, where the doctor put rubber bands on the thumb and forefinger of each of the trainman's hands, and at the same time made firm pressure with his thumb-nails on these ligatured fingers.

The conductor was not informed of the purpose of this procedure, so his imagination had nothing to work on.

After holding his fingers in this manner for

7

about ten minutes the whistle blew, and the conductor had suddenly to leave his chair. He straightened up and went out "on the run."

When he came back he laughed and said: "This is the first time in six weeks I've gotten up or moved without pain. What in thunder have those little rubber bands to do with lumbago, anyway?"

The doctor saw this man before leaving the train two hours afterwards, and the trainman volunteered the information that "so far as the lumbago is concerned I have no more feeling than a fish." And these results can be duplicated by any one who will study the zone charts (Figures 1 and 2), and apply the simple technic outlined.

Naturally, in sciatica, and in articular or joint rheumatism, the results have not been so uniformly favorable. For sciatica may be due to hip joint dislocation. Indeed, one of our most famous bone surgeons claims that all cases of sciatica result from a twist, or subluxation of the hip joint which certainly is not true of those cases cured with a comb, or by electricity, or by some medical measure.

In treating sciatica particular attention must be given the "hip area" of the hand on the same side as the sciatica. This means that the palmar surface of the ring and little finger and the palm of the hand on that side, as well as the "edge" of the palm, running up over the top of the hand must be thoroughly "combed."

But the best and most rapid relief for sciatica is usually secured by "attacking" the soles of the feet — using the comb in the same manner and for the same areas as described for the hands. In other words, by manipulating the zones in the feet corresponding to the zones in the hands.

Dr. George Starr White, of Los Angeles, California, has invented a mechanical device for this purpose, consisting of a piece of hard wood about five inches in length, cut with deep screw-like threads (see Figures 16 and 18). A heavy, smooth rope is attached to each end of this implement of battle, and the patient uses it with a long, strong pull for five or ten minutes at a time — repeating the maneuver several times daily. Possibly any rough-surfaced, home-made device might give equally good results.

In acute articular rheumatism, where there are no gross pathological changes or stiffening in the joints, splendid results have followed the use of combs. It should be remembered that the hip area corresponds with the shoulder on the same side, the knee with the elbow, and the ankle with the wrist, etc., and pain is often overcome more quickly by attacking corresponding parts with pressure or stimulation.

One old lady who suffered terribly in the joints of both hands, and who had not been able to sleep for weeks without an opiate, experienced complete relief after a half dozen treatments with the comb over the tips of her fingers and thumb (Fig. 12). And she was able to sleep soundly thereafter without the use of her usual hypnotic.

A very interesting case of gonorrheal arthritis was reported recently. This man's right knee joint was so painful that he could not bear to have it touched. To bend the right leg at the knee was out of the question.

Two minutes' pressure on the top and bottom, as well as on the tip of the big toe, completely relieved the pain, and upon testing the joint the soreness seemed to have vanished. The doctor then began carefully bending the knee, and to his surprise, and to the amazement of the patient — who hadn't the slightest idea what was being attempted — the knee could be flexed (bent) perfectly, without any pain whatever.

As this doctor makes a specialty of treating painful joints by means of heat, light, mud baths, and electricity, and has had a great deal of experience in this work, we were much gratified to hear him say that of all the cases he had ever treated he never had anything seem so miraculous as this. He further stated that he had tried all his methods of treatment to alleviate this man's pain and to be able to flex the knee, but without avail; yet zone therapy, applied at the proper zone, brought about almost immediate results.

As demonstrating a peculiar phase of zone therapy, and showing how great aches from little corns may grow, here is a very interesting and instructive case. A patient, suffering from rheumatism in the left shoulder and arm, had, for more than three weeks, been unable to sleep on account of the pain. He had a small callous growth on the tip of his left thumb, corresponding to the zone in which the pain was located. This was removed, and pressures were made with a comb on the place where the finger corn had formerly held forth. Within four days he was completely cured.

And this reminds me that a corn doctor is a valuable aid in pressure therapy work. For time and again I have seen pains as far away as a headache relieved by clearing up the zone occupied and irritated by a large pugnacious corn, which was the actual cause of the headache — foolish-sounding as it may seem.

A little boy with an aggravated case of "wry

neck" had, for months, slept upon sand bags to give him neck support. I cauterized the necks of his teeth (always look to the condition of the teeth in wry neck) with a fine platinum point cautery (which is merely a direct way of stimulating all the zones), and in a few days this youngster was up and running around as well as ever.

Other cases of wry neck have been quite as readily cleared up by combing the appropriate fingers on the palm of the hand of the side involved or by pressing with a cotton-tipped probe on the proper zones on the posterior wall of the throat, or on the under surface of the tongue and on the floor of the mouth under the tongue.

Most medical men, without stopping longer than two seconds to think about it, will affirm that all these things are ridiculous and absurd.

This, you remember, was what contemporary scientists told Galen and Harvey, and also what the astronomers told Galileo.

We spoke in a similar strain of radio activity, the fourth dimension, wireless telegraphy, and aerial navigation.

Many erudite members of the medical profession claim that zone therapy and zone analgesia might be interesting if found in Gulliver's Travels or Munchausen's Romances, but that emphatically they have no place in medical literature.   For every one knows that an egg cannot be made to stand on end.

Yet we are standing this medical egg on end every day.

And there is no reason in the world why any intelligent man or woman, let alone any intelligent doctor, cannot do likewise, and put these simple and helpful methods into practical application.   For it doesn't even require faith.

CHAPTER X.

SCRATCHING THE HAND FOR SICK STOMACH.

MANY of us know that if we are threatened with sneezing and we press the upper lip tightly against the teeth with the fingers, that we can usually stop the sneeze. Also, that if we drop a cold piece of metal down the back, or press a piece of ice against the back of the neck, it will frequently check nosebleed.

But not many of us know that the reason these things are thus is because, by these actions, we are stimulating normal function in the first zone.

Were we to press our cheek over the wisdom tooth — which is in the fourth zone — or rub the ice on our third zone ear, the sneeze and the nose bleed would pursue uninterruptedly the even tenor of their ways.

If you never had heard of these things, you would probably say "pish," and look around with some trepidation for your informant's keeper. Yet, in all earnestness and sincerity, I would, if you are one of those whose stomach is easily upset, urge that the next time you board a train or boat you arm yourself with a wire hair brush and a metal comb.

(104)

When the first faint qualms, premonitory of an eruption or some other seismic disturbance in your interior are felt, get busy with the comb and brush — not on your head — but on your hands.

For sickness of the stomach is quite generally relieved by steady pressure made over the first and second zone on the backs of the hands with the teeth of a metal comb. The comb should be pressed firmly over the areas running from the thumb and first finger of both hands, including the web between the thumb and first finger — which seems to have a very intimate connection with the stomach. If there is no comb handy, the finger nails will do good substitute work, but the metal is best, as it seems to stimulate an electrical contact that helps the "impulse."

This procedure is to be used only where the stomach is irritated and threatens convulsive contractures, or where there is pain, or distention from gas. Relief of these conditions may generally be expected in from five to ten minutes.

If, however, the stomach is "dead" — the doctors call it "atonic" — when it lies inert and unambitious after a heavy meal — or even a small meal that is heavy for that stomach at that particular time — the best results are found in gentle stroking or scratching with a wire hair

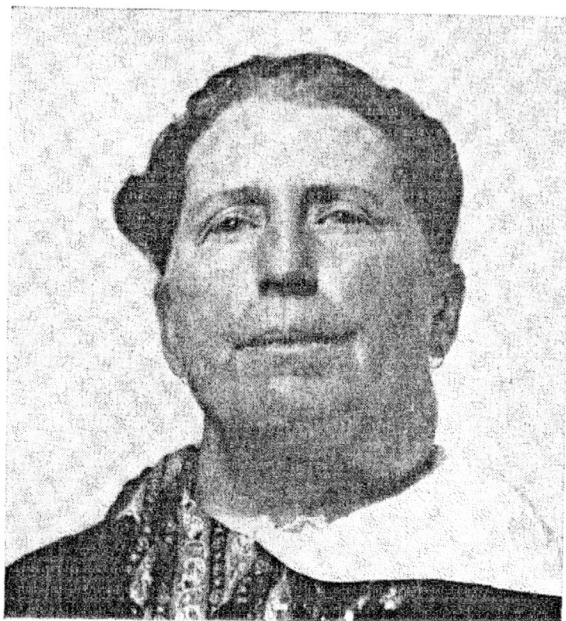

FIG. 21. — When I first saw this patient (January 9, 1913), the enlargement in the neck, pronounced cancer, and inoperable, by some of our best men in New England, was stony hard and exceedingly painful to the touch. She had not been able to lie down for nine months, and had not taken any solid food for three months; could open the mouth only slightly, and with great difficulty. We induced speedy relaxation of the neck (it was absolutely relaxed in four treatments) through pressure with a dry cotton-wound applicator and also with a pencil moistened with trichloracetic acid in varied strengths from twenty-five per cent to a saturated solution, throughout the appropriate zones in the mouth, nose and epipharynx. This patient responds quickly to pressure, and accurately traces sensations of glow or numbness from the mouth to the extremities and vice versa. These sensations are almost immediately followed by lines of anesthesia. Note the neck of this patient (see Fig. 22) fourteen months later. Patient through pressure on fingers of zones involved keeps side of neck constantly anesthetized, and therefore free from irritation, with constant absorption of growth.

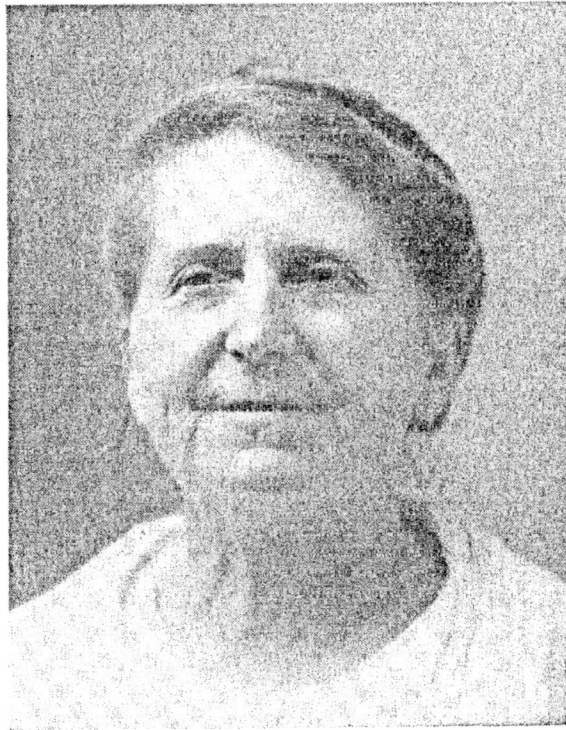

FIG. 22. — Photograph of patient in Fig. 21 seventeen months after her first treatment. After three years improvement still continues.

brush, or with the teeth of the comb. If these are not available scratch with the finger nails, but, as with the pressures, the most favorable results follow the use of metal.

Remember that scratching stimulates, while deep pressure with the teeth of the comb, finger nails or wires of the hair brush relaxes.

Also the next time the baby is restless and inclined to double up and yell murder, instead of doing a slippered constitutional up and down the room with him, scratch the backs of his hands. If he's had too much to eat this may quiet him. If, however, his little "tummy" is "working," try some pressures on his hands or feet, and see how soon the "tummy" will knock off work.

And, for the same sufficient reasons, try the same thing on yourself and the family, instead of "banging" the stomach over the head with a dose of dope.

The morning sickness of pregnancy yields quite uniformly to deep pressures on the backs of the hands, and it is much safer to try and control this nausea from the hands than it would be to resort to the severe pressures on the tongue. For these latter, if too drastic, might produce a miscarriage.

Also, while it isn't exactly zone therapy, it

might be interesting here to note that eating salted popcorn has a tendency to help correct the nausea of pregnancy, car sickness, and indigestion. Many patients of mine keep a bowl of it on a chair right alongside their beds, and commence to eat it so soon as they awake in the morning. A handful of popcorn, thoroughly chewed, seems to help pacify the otherwise rebellious stomach.

Zone therapy pressures are valuable not only in nausea and vomiting, but also in indigestion, gastric catarrh and all forms of stomach disorders. It has even been successfully employed in gastric ulcer, with dangerous hemorrhages and the other distressing symptoms of this painful malady. Dr. Reid Kellogg has cured three of these cases, one in ten treatments, the others in two or three months. Two of these patients had had an acute condition for two months — no food whatosever passing through the pylorus (the exit of the stomach). They had been, of course, fed by the rectum.

Dr. Kellogg used the probe (Fig. 9), low down on the posterior (back) wall of the pharynx, and used pressures over the thumb, first and second fingers of both hands with the aluminum comb.

In less than a dozen treatments these patients

were able to retain food taken into the stomach, and practically conduct the entire subsequent course of their own cure.

To disabuse the minds of any who may evolve the idea that zone therapy is of value only in conditions that "don't matter anyhow," I want to emphasize that these cases were most grave, and that they had received skilled medical attention for many weeks — without apparent benefit.

It has been current knowledge — even before those halcyon days when the banqueter retired to have his throat tickled by a dutiful slave — that by touching definite areas in the throat and at the base of the tongue — vomiting could be induced.

And now we have discovered how to put the reverse English on the tickle, and keep it down when it wants to come up. Which discovery should also help increase the sum total of the world's health and happiness.

CHAPTER XI.

HAY FEVER, ASTHMA AND TONSILITIS.

I F the United States Hay Fever Association, and all individuals who suffer from hay fever, will read carefully, and then apply this chapter—as directed—the ravages of these catarrhal cataclysms, I feel sure, will be beautifully lessened.

For zone therapy has an especial and peculiar message for hay-feverites. It has mitigated, if not entirely relieved, the red-eyed misery of hundreds of them. And none — except those who have been victims — can know what a real relief this is.

Nobody knows for certain what causes hay-fever, and, judging from the textbooks, they know even less regarding any definite method of relieving it.

It is possible that repeated "colds" — generally from dust infection — result in a chronic irritation of the mucous membrane, followed by a thickening (or hypertrophy) of the tissues.

This thickened tissue dams the circulation of blood in the membranes, and presses upon the

delicate nerves of the nose, thereby irritating
them, which irritation proves to be the last straw.
So the nerves of the nose throw up both hands
with a despairing moan.

An acute inflammatory irritation is established, setting up a vicious circle. For the pressure causes nerve irritation, and the nerves re-
taliate by still further disturbing the circulation,
thereby causing more pressure.

Then, if really it is pollen that causes the
physiological conflagration we call hay fever, the
mucous membrane is so susceptible that it will
readily respond to the action of the pollen.
Which is probably also true of those cases that
develop similar conditions from the odor of roses,
horses or cats.

It is significant, however, that of all the hundreds of hay-fever patients that have ever come
under my care not one had an absolutely normal
nose. Invariably there were bony spurs, pro-
truding turbinate bones, cartilages twisted out
of proper alignment, an inflamed and thickened
mucos membrane lining, or some other pathological condition, one usually requiring surgical
interference.

So if you have, or expect to have, hay fever
or any other abnormal condition of the nasal
mucous membranes, see a specialist and have

your nose placed in as near a perfect condition as surgical skill and your physical shortcomings will permit, not forgetting also a thorough stretching of the soft palate. This the surgeon will accomplish by means of a finger inserted in the throat and a hooked instrument in the passage back of the nose. By enlarging the contracted parts of this passage normal drainage and circulation in these tissues is established.

The best results are obtained by operating during the height of an attack. If sometimes even a needle be thrust through the congested mucous membrane, so that the blood flows freely, the attack can be broken up, and the condition frequently eradicated for that season.

Then use any combination of the following procedures, which experience may prove helpful, remembering that here no fixed rule can be laid down, and that what "works" magically in one case might have but little effect in another.

First, make steady firm pressures on various points in the roof of the mouth with the thumb. Be careful to "cover" the region directly on a line with the nose. These pressures should be maintained for from four to eight minutes at a time, and repeated a half dozen or more times daily. Those experienced in zone therapy claim

8

that the pressures have an immediate and powerful effect upon abnormal conditions in this zone.

At the same time the upper lip should be firmly forced against the teeth with the first finger. This usually has a most discouraging effect upon sneezing.

Pressures with a cotton-tipped probe on the back wall of the pharynx (the inside junction of the nose and mouth), as well as upon the mucous membranes of the nose, give, in the hands of physicians, the quickest results. The cotton-tipped probe may be dipped in trichloracetic acid, or some pungent agent, which will lend "punch" to the contact impulse.

A curious feature in connection with this probe therapy is that if the patient, by coughing, resents the presence of the instruments, the effect seems to be dissipated. In other words, the transmission of the nerve impulse is partly inhibited. It is fair to say, however, that patients become rapidly accustomed to what at first frequently caused irritation.

The use of a tongue depressor, covering the center of the tongue fairly well "forward," has also been found most helpful, if pressed down and held firmly several times a day for three minutes or more at a time. In fact, it is expedient to use the tongue depressor in almost all nose, throat and stomach troubles — or, in fact, any condition occurring in the "front" of the body.

The wearing of moderately tight rubber bands upon the thumb, first and second fingers for ten or fifteen minutes (or less, if the finger tips become purple) repeated several times daily, seems also to help materially. Indeed, some physicians report that they get their very best results by having their patients wear the bands as continuously as possible, removing them only as required to prevent blood stasis, and then replacing them again.

Pressures exerted with the finger and thumb over the joints of the thumb, first and second fingers or toes have given excellent results. Three or four-minute pressures with an aluminum comb on all surfaces of the thumb and first finger — repeated several times daily — have also given satisfactory relief in hay fever.

Always the breath should be taken through the nostrils. If the mouth persists in opening at night, strap it shut with isinglass plaster cut in thin strips.

The treatment of asthma and other affections of the respiratory passages is very similar to that of hay fever, excepting that, instead of pressing the tongue, more generally the floor of the mouth is manipulated for this purpose — as the impulse is thus more "direct."

Some of the results in asthma have been little short of miraculous. One patient suffering with bronchial asthma had been unable to lie down for three years, what little sleep she secured being taken propped in a chair. Her sole relief consisted in the hypodermic injection of fifteen drops of adrenalin solution, practically every morning and night.

I made pressure on the pharyngeal wall, at a point "low down," where the "metallic sensation" was reflected into the bronchial region. Also I used the probe on the floor of the mouth, directly beneath the root of the tongue.

Within five minutes this lady — for the first time in three years — was relieved of all pain, tightness, hoarseness, and shortness of breath. In two months of this treatment she gained fifteen pounds, and now sleeps through the night. Also, she has been enabled completely to discontinue her use of adrenalin.

Another bronchial asthmatic suffered so severely that he had made all arrangements, even to packing his trunks, to retire from business and seek health on the Riviera or in Egypt. His "wheezing" was so pronounced that he could be heard clear across a twenty-foot room. This gentleman was advised by Dr. D. F. Sullivan, senior surgeon of St. Francis Hospital, to see me before leaving the country.

I pressed on the floor of the patient's mouth, under the root of the tongue, with a cotton-tipped probe, and made strong pressure on the first and third zones of his tongue with a tongue depressor. In three or four treatments this man was entirely well, and informed us that he had indefinitely postponed his trip abroad, and "was going back to work again."

Zone therapists have found in throat and chest cases that painting the tongue with iodine on the upper and lower surfaces for about one-third way back is most helpful.

But one of the best of all methods by which the patient may help himself consists in biting the tongue as hard as comfortably can be borne, holding that member between the teeth for several minutes at a time, three or four times daily.

Also, it is well carefully to examine the condition of the teeth, throat and pharynx in asthmatic cases, as frequently the asthma does not clear up until some defect in these organs is remedied.

A twelve-year-old girl of my acquaintance, a physician's daughter, has developed considerable technic in zone therapy. Only recently she relieved the pain of a bad case of mumps by fastening spring clothespins to the first, second and third fingers of both her hands, leaving them on until the finger tips became quite purple.

The little lady proudly demonstrated her control over the condition by taking a mouthful of vinegar as a gargle. This, as every doctor knows, is quite a crucial test.

In tonsilitis good results almost invariably follow pressure over the inferior dental nerve, at a point where it enters the jaw bone. It requires considerable skill to find this foramen (as it is called), so this advice is really for doctors only.

Pressure may also be made with the finger on a probe back of the anterior pillars (membranes situated in front of the tonsil).

Yet much may be accomplished merely by squeezing the joints of the second, third and fourth fingers, and using a tongue depressor on the extreme sides of the tongue.

And this reminds me that a certain minister of my acquaintance has been teaching his Boy Scouts zone therapy methods, with especial reference to curing themselves of coughs and other common ailments. The boys also find it valuable in their "First Aid to the Injured" work. I can readily understand that the analgesic effects of zone pressure should be effective in the camp, as well as in the home, or in the dead-of-night emergency.

Zone therapy opens up a tremendous field. So the more experimenters we have the sooner every one will know just how tremendous and useful and marvelous it is.

CHAPTER XII.

CURING A SICK VOICE.

WE all remember the gentleman in one of Moliere's plays who was astounded to learn that he had been talking prose all his life. This verdant reminiscence has an almost universal application.

For instance, Umberto Sorrentino, the gifted Italian tenor, has, for a number of years, relieved the "tight," inflexible throat, which is the bane of vocalists and speakers, by grasping his tongue firmly in a handkerchief, pulling it as hard as could be comfortably borne, and wriggling it slowly from side to side. This, he says, eases up throat tension, and frees the voice. It also has a tendency to abort a beginning cold.

He was led to adopt this practice from observing the beneficial effects of massage of the throat in stimulating and otherwise improving the circulation and releasing the muscles from the bound condition, which invariably (in his case) foreruns a cold. He reasoned that if external massage was beneficial, internal massage should be even more so; hence, the "wriggle."

(120)

Also, Miss Mabel Garrison, one of the new lyric sopranos of the Metropolitan Opera House, has won the appreciation and gratitude of various members of the company, by curing stiff, inelastic sore throats through pressures made upon the vocalists' tongues.

There is a hint in these significant facts that no singer, lawyer, actor, clergyman, mother of a family, or business man can afford to ignore. For almost everyone suffers occasionally from defects somewhere in the delicate mechanism that shapes air currents into beautiful sounds, and molds breath into speech.

Although they probably are not aware of this, both Signor Sorrentino and Miss Garrison are employing zone therapy in relieving these vocal ills. For they are exerting pressures on the first and second zones, the region which governs the function of the vocal chords, the pharynx, larynx, and the respiratory passages.

And while their results have been very remarkable, and eminently satisfactory to themselves and their fellow artists, they would be even more striking were the pressures made more "direct."

In other words, if, instead of squeezing and making strong traction on the tongue, or of using a depressor on this member, they were to

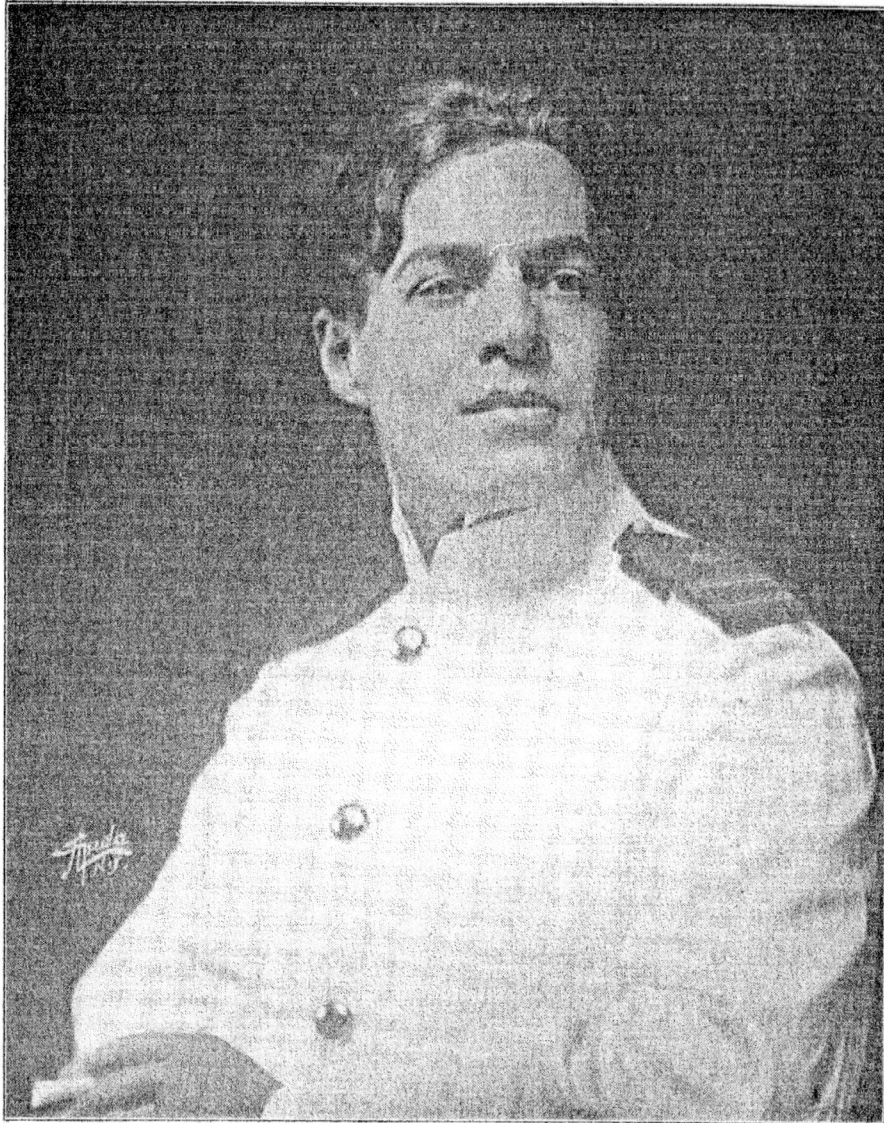

SIGNOR UMBERTO SORRENTINO,

the noted tenor, who relieves "tight" throat by making strong traction on the tongue. By pressure on the anterior third of the tongue, and by stimulating the outside lateral aspects of the fore fingers (which distinctly govern the vocal cords) Sorrentino has relieved himself and many of his friends of what promised to be serious throat conditions.

do these things and, in addition, apply firm pressure on the floor of the mouth, beneath the tongue, with a cotton-tipped metal probe (see Fig. 6), dipped in spirits of camphor or alcohol (to increase the "impulse"), their results would be far more certain and satisfactory.

In all cases of hoarseness, huskiness, or in loss of voice due to irritation or strain — as in clergyman's sore throat — these practices almost invariably give relief. I remember a case of a soprano whose upper register was completely lost through long-continued strain. The floor of her mouth — directly under the tongue, and up to the roots of the lower incisor teeth, was "prodded" intermittently for a period of fifteen minutes, with the metal probe. The cotton on the tip of the probe was dipped in some pungent agent, for the purpose, as before stated, of increasing the nerve "response."

Marked improvement followed the first treatment. She was, however, cautioned not to attempt to use the voice, except for a moment or two after treatments — to observe the effect.

The singer also carried out "home treatments," consisting in five-minute firm applications of a tongue depressor (see Fig. 17) on the center of the tongue. This was done every four hours. In addition, she squeezed the sides of her thumbs. This action, especially if accompanied by digging the finger nails into the inner side of the thumb — which area is distinctly in the vocal chord zone — has a specific effect upon the vocal chords. Within three days this lady had completely recovered, and was able to return to her company.

Zone therapy has, in innumerable instances, restored speaking voices that were as lost as the Lost Hope. Indeed, it is of common occurrence to have a clergyman, a lawyer, or a business man who has become aphonic (voiceless) from long dictation, or some other vocal strain, come to the specialist in zone therapy, unable to speak above a whisper, and within a half hour go his way rejoicing — practically as "good as new".

This, by application of the probe on the floor of the mouth, pressures on the tongue, and sometimes pressures on the thumb and fingers, any and all of which procedures can be successfully used by any intelligent man or woman in the relief of their own troubles, or in curing these troubles in their family.

Respecting the finger pressures, it must be borne in mind that it is necessary to work on the particular zone involved. For instance, it would be useless to make pressures over the thumb joints if the cause of the throat trouble should happen to be a congested tonsil. The third, fourth and fifth fingers would have to be invoked for relief in this zone.

It is, however, perfectly remarkable what these finger pressures alone will accomplish. One of the earlier experimental cases was a patient who had been speaking on and off all day at a Sunday School Convention held in a grove. This grove must have been an ideal spot for a nice open air meeting. But the leafy bowers, the sylvan glades, and the bossy dells were not built for acoustic purposes.

The consequence was that, when the shades of night were falling fast our hero was "all in". He couldn't speak above a whisper. He had such contraction of the muscles that he couldn't even open his jaws — let alone communicate intelligent information through them.

This was his condition when he presented himself the following noon petitioning relief. He had had nothing to eat since late lunch the day before, although, whether he knew it or not, he had had enough then to last him a week.

Of course, as he could not open his mouth it was not possible to treat him by pressures on the floor of the mouth, and on the tongue. So he was provided with an aluminum comb, and shown how to make pressures on the back of his hand, extending up from the thumb to the wrist, and over to the fourth finger, and left to his own devices for twenty-five minutes.

At the expiration of this time he had relaxed the tension of his jaw muscles and relieved the irritation in his throat to such an extent that he went out and had a comfortable lunch. Returning to the specialist's office, pressures were made with a padded probe (see Fig. 9) on the wall of the pharynx — the probe being introduced through the nostril.

Also, he was given instrumentation on the floor of the mouth, underneath the tongue, and a conscientious treatment with a tongue depressor. This weapon he took home and used, carrying out also the combing of the back of the hands. Three days afterwards he sang in the choir as well as ever.

Deep massage with the fingers on the muscles of the throat, and a "plucking" of the voice box are also helpful procedures. Where the irritation or the inflammation is not extensive it might be well to include them as routine measures in most throat troubles. Where there is active congestion they are, of course, not only useless, but actually harmful.

A very frequent cause of vocal ills, and a condition most generally associated with a congested throat, is a "stuffy" nose. Also, it is quite impossible to get a perfect vocal resonance if the membranes of the nose are swollen and congested with "cold" or catarrh.

The tongue and finger pressures do much to relieve these conditions, but perhaps the surest and quickest method of curing them is to "pencil" the nose with a probe, using the uncovered steel for this purpose. And, I may here remark, that the patient's own saliva is one of the best and least irritating lubricants for this probe work in the nose.

The steel should be left in each nostril several minutes, and gently moved back and forth from time to time, for the tonic "penciling" or "ironing" effect. The curative influence of this on chronic nasal catarrh or other pathological conditions of the nose is sometimes quite remarkable.

Also, it might be well here to add that atomizers are useless, except temporarily — as after exposure to a horde of sneezers or coughers. In this event, an alkaline antiseptic may be of value.

But the constant washing away of the natural secretion of the mucous membrane, or the perpetual coating over of the air passages with a film of oil — which prevents the natural secretion from being natural — is distinctly injurious. For it tends to provoke, perpetrate and perpetuate all forms of catarrh, and none should use them — except under physician's instruction — and then for a short time only. Stimulate normal function with a probe or sound, used at night before retiring, and in the morning on arising, and cure the condition instead of making it chronic.

It wouldn't be difficult to get affirmative evidence to the fact that a sick voice is one of the sickest and most disheartening things that can befall one who must depend upon it for a living. But, with a little patience, and an intelligent application of the principles of zone therapy, it is a "cinch".

CHAPTER XIII.

A SPECIFIC FOR WHOOPING AND OTHER COUGHS.

FOR years eminent scientists have been spending much valuable time and money in seeking a cure for whooping cough. Still the whoop persists. The distress, the after effects on the bronchial tubes, and the weakening influence — frequently leading to the later development of tuberculosis — remains uninfluenced. The disease runs its course, irrespective of any or all treatments.

Yet whooping cough is one of the simplest and most easily-cured diseases with which zone therapy has to contend. An ordinary case of whooping cough, which has persisted for weeks, can sometimes be cured in from three to five minutes. Rarely are more than four or five treatments necessary. Case after case is recalled in which, after the application of a cotton-tipped probe — held down firmly on the back of the throat (the post-pharyngeal wall), little patients who had whooped themselves into a state of nervous and physical exhaustion, never had another paroxysm of coughing.

If the savants of the various research institutions throughout the country are really sincere in attempting to discover a cure for whooping cough, asthma, goitre, and a score of other conditions — conditions successfully treated by zone therapy — it will be easy to put this method to the test.

If they do not themselves care to make the experiment, I will come to New York and demonstrate the method on one or one hundred cases, and show that, in from one to a half dozen treatments with a steel probe, whooping cough can be effectively and permanently overcome. This may or may not be worth the attention of these gentlemen. I can do no more than make the offer, which, I emphasize, is made in perfect good faith and in the interest of humanity and science.

The most remarkable feature of a brand-new discovery is very frequently its hoary-headedness. For this reason, when we come to think about this matter of the mechanical relief of cough, we are struck with its antiquity. From time antedating the memory of man, humanity has pressed its second finger in its pharynx (that space which spreads out from the back part of the mouth and throat up into the nose), or the larynx (a continuation of the pharynx), for the purpose of loosening a dry cough or to facilitate expectoration.

All grandmothers, ever since there were grandmothers, have put their fingers in babies' throats to give them relief in croup. Some of the wisest of these grandmothers used to press the handle of a spoon on the back part of the tongue, in order to abort a beginning cold, or cause a profuse secretion of mucous in conditions associated with a dry, metallic cough.

Our old-time cure for hiccoughs has the same reason for its existence. For, when we grasp the tongue of a hiccougher, and with a long pull, a strong pull, and a pull all together, haul the offending member to tongue's length — and hold it there — we cure the spasmodic contraction of the diaphragm (the cause of hiccough) by influencing the zone in which the trouble originates. This is the principle by which we cure whooping cough, or indeed any cough that originates in any portion of the respiratory tube. But, we have found in these cases that spots in the vault or wall of the pharnyx, if pressed firmly with a cotton-wrapped probe, as large as can be comfortably passed through the nostrils, gives the quickest and most definite results.

For the "reflex" — the sensation of pain, tingling, or cold, which is transmitted along the

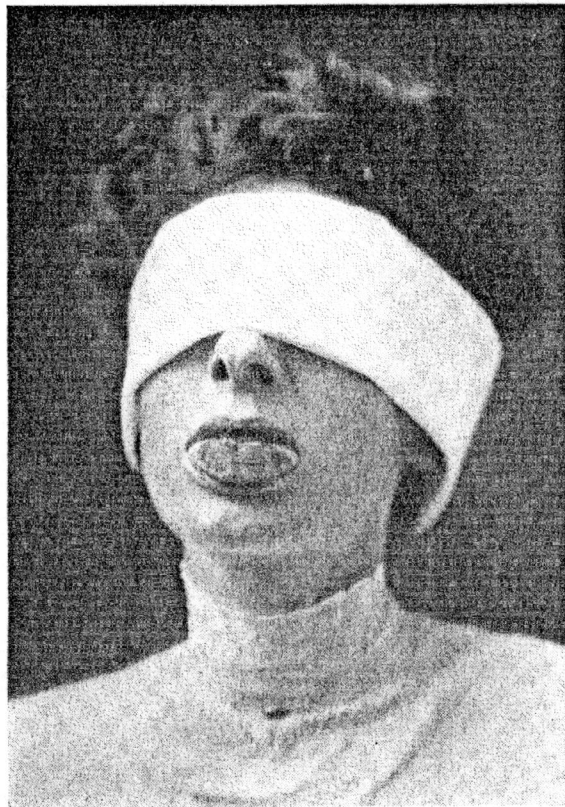

FIG. 23 — Anterior quarter of tongue coated with tincture of iodin
— both surfaces.

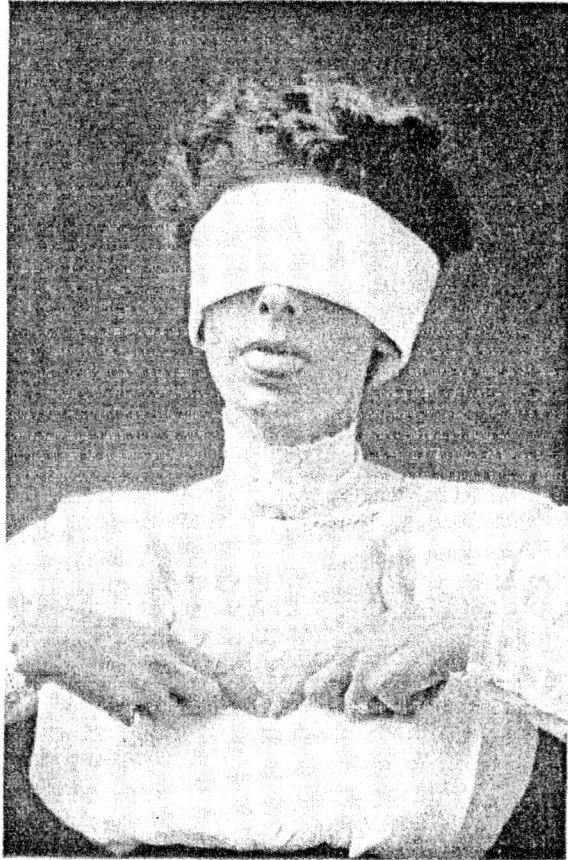

FIG. 24 — Four minutes after complete absorption of the iodin (see Fig. 23) has taken place. The patient is indicating the sensation of heat or reaction over several zones in the chest where it is most pronounced. Few patients experience these sensations, but all patients experience the benefit. This reaction does, as a matter of fact, extend over the entire body. It is easily demonstrated that the tongue, when firmly compressed by the teeth, will often produce relaxation of the entire body, for the mouth is also divided into ten zones. These illustrations indicate the possibility of the speedy absorption of toxins from inner surfaces of neglected teeth and gums.

nerve zones by this contact, — can be definitely traced by the patient to the exact spot where the irritation seems to originate.

By slightly raising the handle of the probe, and thereby altering its point of contact on the business end, this influence can be directed with almost mathematical precision to the area we desire to influence.

When the exact "spot" is pressed—and a little practice will soon make the finding of this almost automatic—the pressure should be firmly held for several minutes. The throat may feel slightly "lame" afterwards — but this soon passes off. If it does not, pressure brought to bear upon the appropriate thumb or finger will relieve the "lameness."

In an experience with several hundred cases of whooping cough we have not yet seen a failure from the proper application of zone therapy. This, I believe, is more than can be truly said of any other form of treatment.

A very few treatments only are necessary to relieve even the most aggravated case of whooping cough—or any cough which originates in the respiratory passage in that zone.

In other words, a tubercular cough, which has its cause in a lesion on the extreme right or left of the lung would not respond to pressures in the middle zones. Likewise a cough which was reflected from a congested liver, or from some other organ not in the first and second zones, would fail to respond to pressures made as here described. Any intelligent man or woman can apply these pressures — and with almost the same success as would attend the effort of the most famous specialist.

It sometimes assists very materially if the tongue, for about a third way back, is thoroly painted above and below with tincture of iodin. The mild irritation from the iodin tends to stimulate the normal function of all those zones interested in keeping up the cough.

If the use of the probe through the nostrils seems too much like a surgical operation, very good—though not so rapid and effective results —will follow the application of firm pressures on the front part of the tongue, and on the floor of the mouth directly under the tongue.

Also moderately tight rubber bands should be worn on the thumbs and first fingers of both hands for five or ten minute intervals, several times a day. This might be supplemented also with strong pressure with the finger and thumb over the bridge of the cougher's nose.

If there should be a frontal headache associated with the cough—a very frequent symptom if the cough has persisted for any length of time—the finger and thumb should be moved up to the very root of the nose. This shall be pinched gently for several minutes, right at the place where the nose ends and the eyes begin.

One of the most remarkable things zone therapy has yet done (although I am not surprised at anything it may do) was to cure a forty-year-old cough, originating in a tracheal (or wind pipe) irritation. The patient received one treatment with a probe (Fig. 9) on the back wall of the pharynx.

She experienced relief after the second treatment, and continued to improve until, at the expiration of three weeks, she was discharged as cured. Now, after 15 months, there has been no return of the cough.

Another patient with bronchial cough associated with lagrippe, under my instruction, relieved herself by pressures made with the finger and thumb over the bridge of the nose, and by the wearing of rubber bands around the thumbs and first fingers of both hands.

This lady reported the following morning that she had enjoyed the first night's sleep she had had in more than five nights, and that a persistent and most annoying headache had also cleared up.

These results are quite uniform, and can be duplicated by any one who will try patiently and painstakingly to duplicate them.

Indeed, so simple is the procedure that I have repeatedly seen bronchial and other coughs, resulting from irritation or congestion at some point in the air passages, completely cured, merely by pressure on the tongue with the handle of a tablespoon or a toothbrush. And many of these had persisted for a long time.

I believe the time is not far distant when every one will be his own cough doctor; when mothers, instead of doping their children with dangerous opiates or stomach-destroying nostrums will, with a tongue depressor, or a probe, do successfully in a few hours what now (to perpetrate an Irish bull) is done inadequately or not at all in many days.

Here is the knowledge. There are no patents or restrictions upon it. Every one is free to use it to the fullest and most helpful possible extent.

CHAPTER 14.

HOW A PHANTOM TUMOR WAS DISSIPATED.

LAST June the New Hampshire Dental Society held a convention at Weirs, on Lake Winnepesaukee. One of the residents of the summer colony was brought before the convention on the evening of June 23d. Her serious condition baffled the local physicians. It was hoped that among the two hundred scientific men, gathered there from all parts of the East, some might be found who could help her.

She was a woman about thirty-five years old, well nourished and apparently healthy, apart from a large swelling in the front of the neck. Manifestly the thyroid and other glands had become enlarged through some unknown inflammatory cause. She was suffering great pain. The slightest touch caused agony. Swallowing was impossible. Not even a drop of water had passed down her throat since the preceding Friday night. This was Wednesday night.

A healthy human being can exist from seven to ten days without water. This woman had been without water for five days, suffering mental and physical torture. Her physician insisted, as the only means of saving her life, that an operation be performed at once. The half dozen or more physicians who had been called in consultation concurred in this. There was nothing left but to perform an intubation — the insertion of a tube in the gullet, through which water and food might be passed, pending some possible measure of relief.

The heart was racing along at one hundred and fifty beats a minute, and there were all the peculiar symptoms usually associated with thyroid disturbances. Inasmuch as the whole trouble had developed in a week, it was most unlikely that the condition was goitrous.

As it was probable that the trouble was associated with the thyroid, a physician present decided to try zone therapy, because it could be applied instantly, and promised immediate results if successful.

Calling one of the dentists to make strong pressure over the first joint of one thumb, the doctor grasped the other thumb. This simple, apparently foolish, treatment was maintained for three minutes. The patient began to show signs of relief. The drawn lines on her face softened. She could bear without shrinking the touch on her neck.

The doctor sent for a glass of water, and held

it to the patient's lips. She took a sip of water, which she swallowed with much difficulty and pain — the first drop in five days.

"It is the most delicious thing I ever tasted," she whispered.

She was able to swallow about a third of a glass upon her first attempt. The pressures were continued intermittently for about an hour, and within that time she was able to drink four glasses of water and a glass of malted milk. A light rubber band was placed over her thumb joints, as shown in Fig. 5, and she enjoyed her first night's sleep since the inflammation had developed.

The next morning she reported that she was almost entirely relieved. The swelling was hardly perceptible, and she could bear reasonable pressure over the glands without discomfort. She had no difficulty in swallowing. In a few days she was fully recovered, and has had no return of the trouble.

With the relief of nerve tension—consciously or unconsciously exerted—there necessarily follows a relief in either the constricted or the congested condition of the lymphatic glands or ducts, the thyroid and other ductless glands, and also of the vasomotor nerves, which control the flow of blood through the blood vessels.

This action, no doubt, accounts for the marvelous results which zone therapy has produced in the treatment of glandular and circulatory diseases — whether due to nervous, or physical causes.

In the famous "globus hystericus"—that big lump comes up in the throat of an hysteric— there is no speedier or more effective treatment than zone therapy. Merely take the hands of the hysterical individual, squeeze them as hard as she can bear the pressure, and maintain this pressure for several minutes. Almost immediate relaxation of all the zones will follow, and with this relaxation a disappearance of the great lump in the throat.

The combs or the wire hair brush may be used, if preferred. Or, if none of these are available, merely scratch the back of the hands with the finger nails. It will help materially, of course, if suggestion be employed, using the voice in a soothing manner.

But the results are quite as effective — although not as rapid—if the patient has no idea concerning what is being attempted.

CHAPTER 15.

DR. WHITE'S EXPERIENCE.

ONE of the most thoro and able diagnosticians in America, if not in the world, is George Starr White, M. D., of Los Angeles, Cal., discoverer of the bio-dynamic method of diagnosis. I reproduce a small portion of his experiences in zone therapy and zone anesthesia—as detailed in his Lecture Course.

"A few years ago, while experimenting on the anesthetic effect of the Tesla current, I observed that by giving a current that produced a severe shock to the fingers, I was able to pierce them with needles and not feel pain. I did not realize why these results were obtained. But experiments on animals gave me a hint. For one of my horses backed into a window, and got a large piece of glass into the sacral region (near the tail). We tried, without success, to put her into a narrow stall and tie her legs so we could operate, as a large incision had to be made to extract the foreign body. Finally one of our men suggested that we tie a slipper-noose, which he called a 'twitch', around the horse's nose. He made this 'twitch' out of a piece of thin rope, put it on the horse's nose, and we started to operate. The result was a collision between the horse's hind legs and my abdomen. I told the man to put the 'twitch' on again, tie it tightly, and hold it for two or three minutes. Then, altho I made a deep incision to take out the glass, the horse did not flinch.

"I realize now that we used zone anesthesia, as the sacral region and the nose are in the same zone. At other times we have had occasion to do minor operations on cows and pigs on my experiment farm, and have noticed that, by putting a 'twitch' on the nose, the animals did not seem to experience any pain.

"Also, before anesthesia was so well known, I remember seeing surgeons do minor operations on individuals who would take no chloroform. Almost always the patients closed their teeth, or clinched their hands on some rough substance. Then 'they could stand anything.'

"Later I heard Dr. William H. Fitzgerald explain zone therapy. Then I realized that we have always used zone therapy, although we did not know it.

"After spending a few days with Dr. Fitzgerald, I met at a dinner party, a lady who had a severe frontal headache. Obtaining her permission to try a new 'cure', I exerted pressure upon the thumb, first and second fingers, and within five minutes the headache had disappeared. I had similar success in treating a toothache.

"I shortly afterwards called on a New York physician who had previously been one of my pupils, and asked him if he knew anything about zone therapy. He said he did not, but had read about it in some of the journals, and thought 'it must be all imagination.' I then held his fingers, pretending I was trying to see how much resistance there was in his muscles. Within three minutes I laid a button hook on his eyeball without his flniching. I took a stickpin from his cravat, and pushed it into his cheek, and put several pins into his face, without his feeling them. He could not bear the touch of a pin in any other zone. He called his wife, and she was horrified when she saw him so 'stuck up.' I withdrew the pins and sterilized his face. He is now a staunch believer in zone anesthesia.

"At several of our lecture courses in Chicago and elsewhere, I had an opportunity to show these methods, and made some very interesting observations. We found that light would not contract the pupil of the eye that had been attacked through the finger zones to the same degree as the pupil of the eye that had not been so attacked.

"One of the doctors in a Chicago class, on hearing of zone anesthesia, told me that about two years previous he was suffering from inguinal hernia (rupture) and a radical operation was advised. He went to the hospital, and the anesthetist began to prepare him for the anesthesia. He told them that he wanted no anesthesia, as he was going to have the operation done without taking anything. The surgeon was loath to operate without some kind of general or local anesthetic, but he told him he wanted nothing, as he thought he could control himself. The surgeon consented, but had ready chloroform and a hypodermic with cocaine. The Doctor clinched his teeth and hands with all his might, and put himself into as powerful a tension as possible for about three minutes before lying on the table. He then laid down, relaxed, and said 'go ahead.' From the beginning to the end of the operation all he noticed, he said, was that there was something going on, but he felt absolutely no pain. I looked at his teeth, and saw that the occluding (biting) surfaces were very good indeed, which accounts in a great measure for the efficacy of the zone anesthesia.

"Dr. Fitzgerald has treated many cases of

10

cancer and tumor, and has had some extraordinary successes with some of them. He carefully avoids any reference to the value of zone therapy in these conditions, but, to my mind, the results achieved warrant mention. I saw two most interesting cases in his practice. One, a lady, about 55 years of age, had a growth on the side of her neck, diagnosed as cancer. By the biodynamic method, I confirmed this diagnosis. This growth was as large as an ordinary sized orange, and very hard and unyielding. The lady told us that, until she began being treated by means of zone therapy and zone analgesia, she had not slept for months without some opiate. For more than two years now she said she had taken no opiates, and had rested without any pain when zone pressure anesthesia was used.

"When I saw this lady the size of the growth had diminished from this treatment, until it would not be recognized except by palpation (feeling with the fingers). I also saw her photograph, taken before she began treatment, and the improvement was certainly remarkable. I do not know whether zone therapy will ever cure this case, but we do know that it is making life endurable to the unfortunate victim.

"Several of my pupils have used the Fitzgerald method for operation on turbinate and other nasal obstructions, as well as upon obstetric (childbirth) cases, with most gratifying results in all of them.

"Two or three cases out of ten will not, it seems, respond to zone therapy. But the majority will. There is no doubt a good reason for the failures, such as blocking of the 'zone paths' in some manner—as by a tumor, growth, pus condition, or obstruction. Or again, failure may be due to faulty technic. Better results will no doubt come with more experience. It only requires that the method be tried out on a huge scale, and by a large number of competent observers. Then the collated results will furnish us a basis for accurate application of these most wonderful and helpful principles."

CHAPTER 16.

ZONE THERAPY — MAINLY FOR DENTISTS.

THERE are four reasons why zone analgesia—as we call the pain-relieving properties of zone therapy—are not more generally used by dentists. One is that the dentist doesn't wish to put himself in the embarrassing position of suggesting such a foolish-seeming thing to his pain-racked patient. Another is that the patient herself thinks she's conferring a favor upon the dentist by permitting him to spend five or ten minutes' valuable time in attempting to alleviate her sufferings, and make the ordeal of cavity preparation or scaling comparatively painless.

Also, to press over the roots of a tooth for three, four, or more minutes—exerting, after toleration is established, all the force of which the operator is capable—is hard work. It's much quicker and easier, and less likely to numb the dentist's thumb and finger, to "slap" a gas cone over the patient's nose, or inject cocaine around the gums—which, to my mind, hurts almost as badly as having the tooth extracted.

(148)

There is yet another reason, however, which partially justifies the previous three. The analgesic results of zone pressure are not sufficiently uniform to "bank" on. In other words, a dentist, led by previous successes, might be tempted confidently to assure a patient of the painlessness, under zone analgesia, of a certain operation. But when he commenced to work he might almost lift the top of his victim's head off. To obviate this do not limit the pressure to three minutes only, and do not attempt to operate or extract until a puncturing test with a sharp instrument shall prove the part to be desensitized.

Also, I would here emphasize that there is no use in attempting, with zone analgesia, to relieve pain if it is desired to remove a nerve. We do not pretend to explain why it is possible, for instance, to work thirty-five minutes, (as demonstrated before the Mass. Dental Society by Dr. B. A. Sears, of Hartford) and cut the jaw bone all to pieces in order to remove an impacted wisdom tooth, while we are unable to thrust a nerve broach into a root canal. But the fact remains, and some time, when pathologists and other experts have studied these problems, we may know why. But for the present, we must be content to be guided by dearly-bought experiences.

There is no known way of telling in advance, just what degree of analgesia success is assured. Dr. M. W. Maloney, of Providence, R. I., and Dr. Wm. J. Hogan, of Hartford, Conn., claim successful results with about 80% of their cases. Dr. Everett M. Cook, of Toledo, Ohio, writes that he is easily successful in 75% of his cases. Dr. Thomas J. Ryan, of New York, is quite uniformly successful in desensitizing the gums for pyorrhoea treatment. While other dentists range on down to as low as 50% of successes, or even to zero.

There are probably very definite reasons for this, although it may be difficult to convince the average dentist that such exist. First, it requires a fine technic to find the various dental nerves, and, by commencing gently, and gradually increasing pressures, to anesthetize them without hurting the patient more than the operation might have hurt him. In which case he has the pain of the operation plus the pain of attempting to analgesize his unresponsive nerve points.

Next, when pressures are made over the fingers, especially where no clamps or rubber bands are used, there is a tendency to skimp on the time devoted to the finger squeezing. The dentist or his assistant will give the job a "lick and a promise"—and let it go at that. They don't use sufficient time or sufficient force really to accomplish anything.

And third, they won't take the time properly to learn the zones and the teeth relations, and apply in a serious way the knowledge so acquired.

However, for the benefit of those dentists who may be interested in learning how to desensitize cavities in sensitive teeth, or do some of the necessarily painful scaling of tartar and other deposits in pyorrhea, and for the particular benefit of several million of their patients throughout the country, I would say that pressure by an assistant exerted over the joints of the thumb (the assistant would do better completely to "cover" the joint, using thumbs and fingers of both hands for this purpose), will mitigate or quite control the pain in the incisor and occasionally the cuspid teeth of the side corresponding to the finger being squeezed.

Never let the patient do this for himself, unless you provide him with clamps or wide rubber bands for the purpose, as he cannot be trusted to make the pressures long enough or strong enough to accomplish satisfactory results.

Pressure exerted over the first or second joint of the first finger will control pain in the cuspid and bicuspid teeth. The second finger is related to the two molars, but sometimes the third (or ring) finger must also be employed for this region.

In other words, pressure upon the thumb, fore-finger, middle, and ring fingers of either hand will control correspondingly pain in the incisors, cuspids and bicuspids and the two molars on either side of the median line, providing that there is no great inflammation or no abscess in the vicinity of the corresponding teeth.

Occasionally the "control" over-laps, in which case it it necessary to use also the finger next to the zone finger, and in the case of wisdom teeth, to get the best results it is sometimes advisable to use both the third and the little finger —as the fourth and fifth zones merge in the head.

A very successful method practiced by some experts—particularly where extraction must be done — is to grasp the offending tooth as near the apex of the root as is practicable, and with the thumb and finger make firm pressure for three, four, or more minutes — by the watch. This usually produces a degree of anaesthesia lasting about one half hour, although pressure can, if necessary, be reapplied at any time.

Other dentists and oral surgeons get excellent

results by pressing on the "heel of the jaw"—
the point directly back of the wisdom tooth,
ponderously known as "the tuberosity of the
superior maxillary." This produces a very complete and lasting anaesthesia of the entire jaw

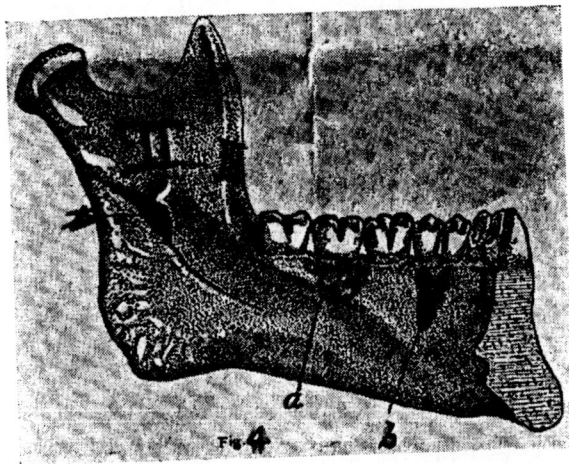

FIG. 25 — Pressure at I, Fig. 4, with thumb and finger will anesthetize
both thumb zones, inasmuch as the pressure is brought directly on the
median line and to the right and left of it.
  Pressure at II (pressure on inferior dental and lingual nerves) will
anesthetize not only entire jaw on side compressed, but to a greater or
less extent the entire half of the body.
  Pressure at a with thumb and finger will often anesthetize that zone
sufficiently for painless extraction. Any tooth may be prepared similarly.
  Pressure at b with thumb and finger anesthetizes bicuspids and occasionally molars.
  Pressure at III will aid materially in anesthetization.

of the side affected, and permits of the painless
extraction of teeth living in the immediate
neighborhood.

With the lower front teeth, it has been found
that to press or hold the inferior (or lower)

dental nerve, where it enters the ramus (or groove) of the lower jaw, gives good anaesthesia. Also pressure with the finger on the inferior dental nerve, where it exits from below the bicuspid tooth (called by doctors the mental foramen) will usually anesthetize that half of the jaw.

Many operators, the better to "focus", prefer to use the blunt end of an instrument (the handle of an excavator is excellent) upon this inferior dental nerve.

The proper application of these principles cannot fail to be of immense value to the dentist and oral surgeon in their daily practice. In relieving toothache and neuralgia, in removing deposits, in extracting teeth, and in fact in most painful operations which dentists are called upon to perform, this pressure technique should prove invaluable, as many dentists are learning every day.

And further, the application of these principles will inevitably encourage public interest in dentistry, and will materially diminish the sum total of pain and suffering that humanity is called upon to endure. Indeed, it is common —and highly gratifying—among many dentists now using zone analgesia—to have sensitive patients—those upon whom, because of past exhausting and nerve-racking experiences, they have always dreaded working—say "Well, Doctor, if you never hurt me any more than you did today I shall never again fear to come to you."

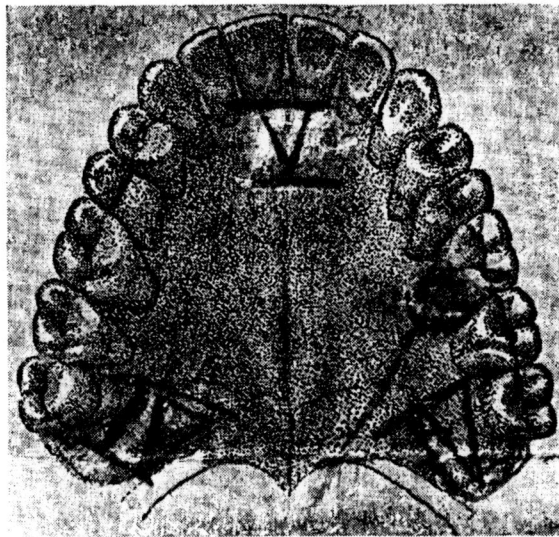

FIG. 26 — Pressure at IV will not only anesthetize the third and fourth zones, but frequently also that half of the upper jaw.

Pressure at V with finger covering the median line and counter pressure with the thumb on the outside of the jaw, or even on the lip directly opposite the finger, will usually anesthetize the incisors sufficiently for painless extraction.

Mothers will find this method a safe and certain means of relieving themselves and their children of an immense amount of pain and discomfort. For, while they cannot, of course, hope to possess the technical knowledge enabling them to find and exert pressure upon the nerves themselves, it is a comparatively simple matter for them to rigidly grasp the roots of an aching tooth between their thumb and finger, and temporarily relieve pain—at least until they can take little Alfred or Alice to the dentist.

If this may not seem feasible, they can, by remembering the fingers that correspond with the particular zone it is desired to influence, do much to relieve distressing conditions in that zone until such time as the doctor or dentist can be visited, by squeezing, or by applying rubber bands around the proper fingers.

For example: At a dinner party the other night one of the guests complained of severe pain in the right upper first molar. I told her to squeeze firmly the joint of her second or middle finger, which advice she considered a very ill-timed and pointless joke. Insisting that I was serious and helpfully disposed, she obeyed instructions, and in a very few minutes beamed complete relief from her dental anguish.

Another instance in which toothache was relieved in what might be called an *outre'* manner was reported by Dr. J. F. Roemer of Waukegan, Ill., who operated with a pair of rubber bands upon the aching teeth of a young traveling man. Dr. Roemer writes that this man came to the office with an extremely painful and sensitive condition, chiefly affecting the incisor teeth. As the knight of the leather bag explained it his teeth were so "sore" that he could not eat any solid food whatever, and he didn't much relish the food he drank. It was impossible for him to close his teeth together without causing great distress. A dentist who had examined the salesman could find nothing wrong with the teeth, from the dental standpoint.

Dr. Roemer, however, examined him in a characteristic zone therapy way. He searched the patient's fingers with a metal comb to find out what was the matter with his teeth. This search disclosed the presence of "spots" on the insides of the thumb and first finger which were acutely sensitive to pressures from the teeth of the comb.

The diagnosis established, the treatment was simplicity itself. Commencing with light pressures upon these sensitive areas the doctor gradually increased the force applied to the comb, at the same time engaging the owner of the thumb and teeth in conversation relative to his business, and to the political situation—this latter a perennial source of interest-absorbing conversation in the West.

After about ten minutes of this operation the doctor looked up and asked his victim "how the

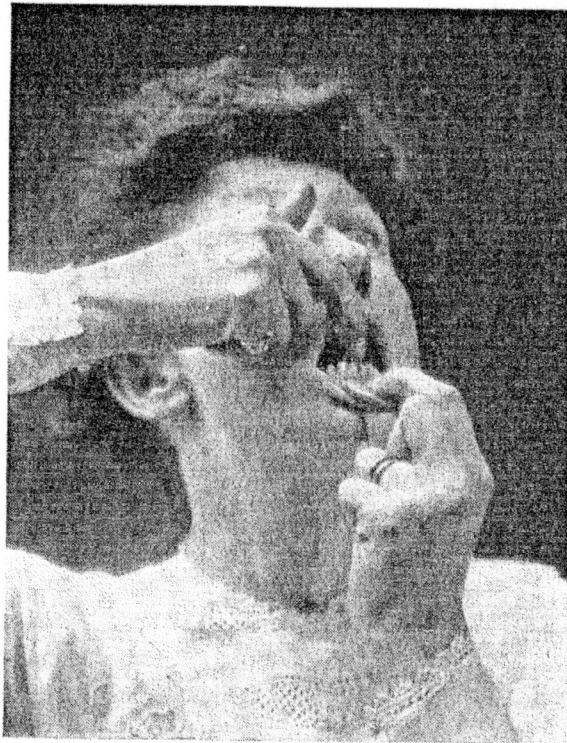

FIG. 27 — Patient anesthetizing the left jaws in the first zone, by firmly pressing the lip directly opposite, between the thumb and index finger of left hand, indicating the area with the right index finger.

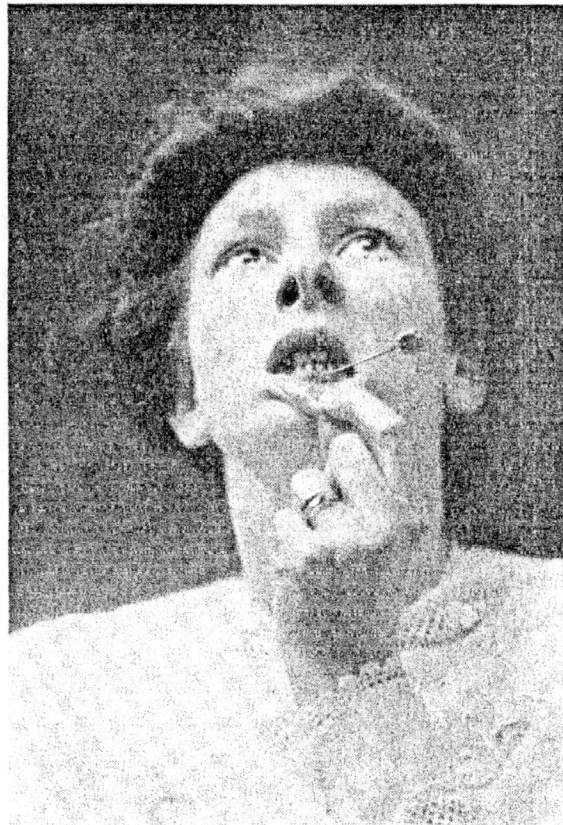

FIG. 28 — Stickpin firmly imbedded in a section of the anesthetized area shown in Fig. 27.

teeth were getting along." After cautiously testing their sensitiveness by means of various biting pressures, the patient responded that "while they were still a little 'sore' the pain had entirely left."

The doctor then issued instructions as to how to apply rubber bands in order to make the proper pressure, which is to use one-fourth inch bands about two inches in length, bind them around the first joint—counting from the tip—of the thumb and first finger, leave them on until bluish discoloration appeared, then remove, and re-apply after a few hours.

The traveling-man reported the following day that he had enjoyed a good night's sleep—the first for many nights — and after forty-eight hours of this treatment he telephoned that all pain and sensitiveness had completely disappeared.

In neuralgia and other painful conditions of long standing, where there are no decayed teeth —or other dental causes for the pain—many permanent cures have been effected by pressure treatment. Almost it would seem that whatever tends to reduce the pain would also help remedy its cause, no matter how remote.

As illustrating, in detail, the successful "home treatment" of neuralgia, another case of Dr.

Roemer's is most interesting. The Doctor says "I saw recently a patient with tri-facial neuralgia of two years' standing. Nothing had relieved permanently. The attack which brought him to me was of four or five days' duration. During this time he had been unable to eat. Even the attempt to speak would bring on an acute paroxysm of pain of a sharp piercing nature, which radiated over the entire left side of the face, extending from the lower and the upper jaw, and up into the left eye. These paroxysms left him as 'limp as a rag.'

"He had been advised to have the nerve cut, as offering the only relief for his trouble.

"I applied rubber bands on the joints nearest the tip of the thumb and forefinger of the left hand. In less than ten minutes my patient was talking and laughing, and we had quite a visit.

"I told him nothing about what was being attempted with the bands, so he wasn't 'hypnotized.' After we saw results, however, I instructed him to apply the bands every half hour if the pain continued, and as it decreased to lengthen the interval of the applications.

"When next I saw him, several days after, he laughingly said, 'Oh, I apply the rubbers once a day now, as I don't want that pain to come back.' He is now enjoying life better than he has for

11

years, thanks to 'those fool rubber bands,' as his daughter called them."

Many dentists secure a very satisfactory degree of analgesia — sufficient for excavating or treatments—by compressing firmly the lip or cheek immediately over the tooth that is to be worked upon. (See Fig. 27.) But as a rule, for extraction purposes, they prefer pressure over the roots, or directly upon the various branches of the dental nerves. (See Figs. 25 and 26.)

One of the most significant facts in connection with zone therapy is the intimate relation between morbid dental conditions and pain or even pathological changes in practically every section of the body. It has been demonstrated beyond a shadow of doubt, that points—or foci —of infection within the mouth, or in the teeth, frequently manifest disturbances most remote from their point of origin.

This is one reason why many physicians and surgeons, using the method, make a routine practice of sending every patient, in whom dental disease is even suspected, for a thorough overhauling by a competent dentist.

Another reason for striving to keep all our original teeth in their places is that nature intended to preserve the continuity—if it may be so termed—of our various nerve zones. Sound, healthy teeth and roots in their normal occlusion, seem to assist in the normal functioning of the entire zone chain of which they are important links.

Asthma, congestions, headaches, neuralgia, conditions affecting the nerves of the head or the ears, or even partial deafness, have been materially improved, and many times completely cured, by the application of a galvanic cautery around the necks of the teeth, by pressure on the teeth themselves in the zone affected, or even by having the patient "grind" the particular teeth related to those areas which it is attempted favorably to influence.

In several instances, chronic frontal headaches in children have been cured by correcting faulty occlusion of the front teeth by that branch of dentistry known as "Orthodontia." When after several months' treatment, the teeth were restored to their normal alignment, and continuity of the nerve zone was re-established, the headaches cleared up, and there has been no return of them.

Occasionally it happens that a patient will go to a physician who uses zone analgesia to be prepared for the services of a dentist who doesn't. Only recently a man suffering from indigestion

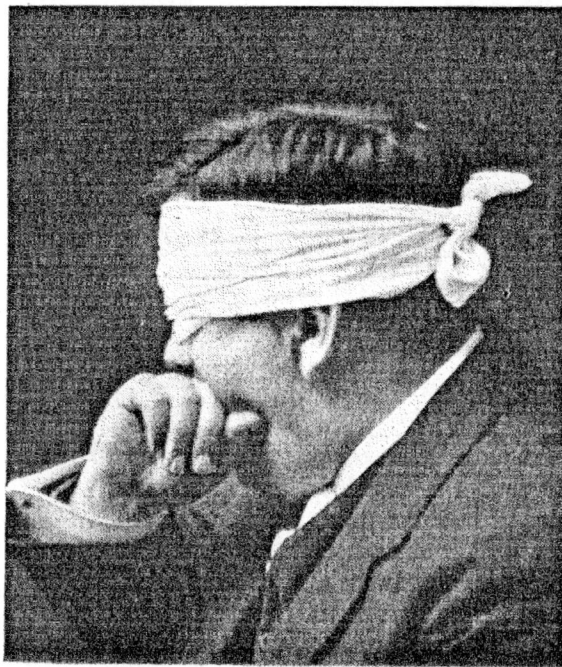

FIG. 29 — A prominent Connecticut dentist anesthetizes the entire left half of his body through pressure on left inferior dental nerve. See following cut.

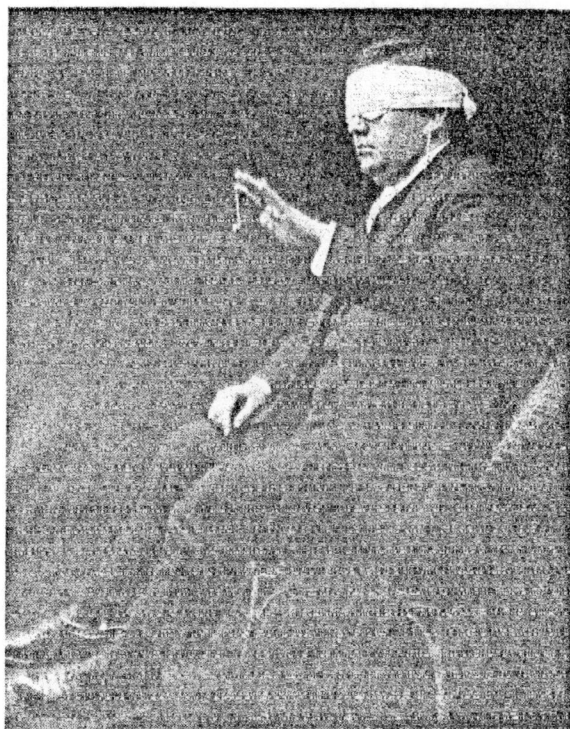

FIG. 30.—We might have covered the left side of the body with stickpins without his knowledge, as far as pain was concerned, during the period of fifteen minutes of anesthesia which followed his pressure of one minute with the finger on the left inferior dental nerve. Note the stickpins in ear, finger and leg.

and rheumatoid arthritis (rheumatism of the joints with progressive stiffening) was advised by his physician to have his teeth removed, the doctor insisting that because four wisdom teeth were the only teeth he had that were not decayed and completely broken down, nothing else would cure his indigestion and rheumatism.

His heart action was such that it would have been dangerous to administer cocaine — much less a general anesthetic.

Therefore, for the removal of his 27 teeth and stumps, the pressure method was decided upon. His physician accompanied him to the dentist, and doctor and dentist, for the next twenty minutes made the proper pressures on the fingers and on the inferior dental nerves.

All the lower teeth were then removed—without a particle of pain. Pressures were then repeated on the fingers and the palatine nerves, and the teeth in the upper jaw were likewise removed.

Of the entire 27, only two gave much pain on extraction, and these were most strongly attached to the bony processes (the sockets and attachments by which teeth are held in place). Bleeding following this wholesale extraction was very slight.

It may be interesting to know that after the gums had healed and the patient had worn artificial teeth for a few months, his appetite and digestion improved, he began to gain in weight, and there was an almost complete relief from the rheumatic symptoms and the joint stiffening.

In some instances physicians have applied the pressures in their own offices, and have then sent the patients — with rubber bands bound tightly around their finger joints in order to maintain the analgesic influence—to the dentist, where their extraction or cavity preparation has been painlessly done.

And occasionally great pleasure and satisfaction is afforded both patient and doctor when some sufferer calls up on the 'phone at two or three in the morning and inquires what finger to press to relieve the pain of a certain tooth, especially when the advice given has been followed by relief.

It has been for many years a quite general piece of knowledge among dentists that the application of menthol to the mucus membrane of the nose, on the same side as an aching tooth, would very frequently stop the toothache. If dentists will now apply a slight elaboration of this bit of zone analgesia technic they may pos-

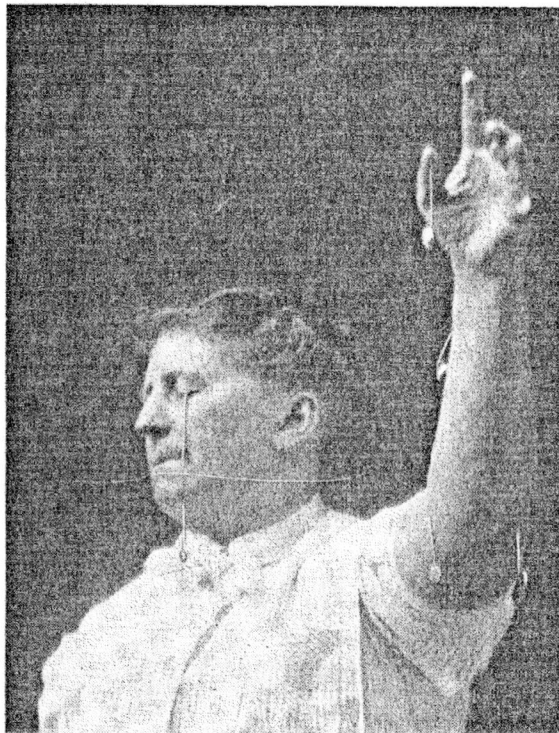

FIG. 31 — Hand and arm, left eyelid and chin, decorated with stickpins after the patient has anesthetized the left side of the body by pressure on the left inferior dental nerve.

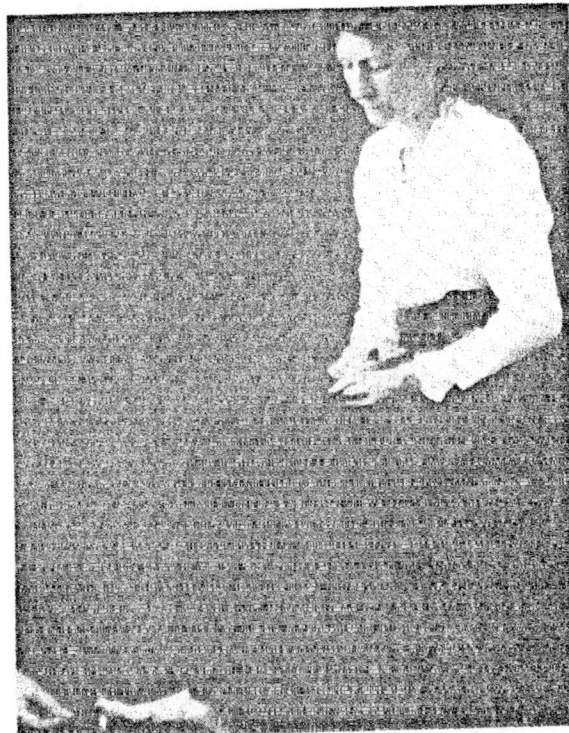

FIG. 32 — A lighted match is held beneath patient's right great toe, anesthetized through pressure on the inner surface of the jaw in the first zone.

sibly save themselves many gray hairs. What their patients will save in agony, apprehension, and the drain on their vitality cannot be even estimated.

CHAPTER 17.

ZONE THERAPY — FOR DOCTORS ONLY.

WE grind and grit our teeth during paroxysms of pain. When we bump our shins against a rocking-chair that has taken point of vantage directly in our path, immediately we clasp the offended shin.

In the days before the blessed era of nitrous-oxid and local anesthetics, when the muscular dentist leaned toward the door with our pet tooth in the firm embrace of shiny forceps, we helped him to the utmost by gripping the arms of the chair with vise-like clutch. This maneuver seemingly had no more connection with tooth extraction than have the effulgent rays of the moon upon the pumpkin crop. But we felt our duty, and we did it.

When fury and anger sweep us in their red flame, and gentle, familiar aspects of nature take on the hue of blood, we clench our fists until the nails are driven deep into the flesh. In the first shock of the agony of bereavement, or during those cruel dragging hours when we are adjusting ourselves to living with our hearts torn asunder, we clasp our hands in frenzy.

(171)

For ages we have been doing these things because they are natural and apparently inevitable. We did them automatically, without knowing why. But now we know we do them because they are instructive and scientific. We do these things involuntarily and automatically because they relieve pain or nerve tension—because they produce a form of analgesia, or pain-deadening, similar to that which follows the injection of water or some anesthetic solution into a sensory nerve.

Six years ago I accidentally discovered that pressure with a cotton-tipped probe on the muco-cutaneus margin (where the skin joins the mucus membrane) of the nose gave an anesthetic result as though a cocaine solution had been applied.

I further found that there were many spots in the nose, mouth, throat, and on both surfaces of the tongue which, when pressed firmly, deadened definite areas to sensation. Also, that pressures exerted over any bony eminence, on the hands, feet, or over the joints, produced the same characteristic results in pain relief. I found also that when pain was relieved, the condition that produced the pain was most generally relieved. This led to my "mapping out" these various areas and their associated connections, and also to noting the conditions influenced through them. This science I have named zone therapy. It is somewhat complicated in many of its aspects, but I shall try and make it as clear as may be. I would emphasize, however, that to master it requires long study and patient application.

In zone therapy we divide the body longitudinally into ten zones, five on each side of a median or central line. (See Figs. 1 and 2.) The first, second, third, fourth and fifth zones begin in the toes and end in the thumbs and fingers, or begin in the thumbs and fingers and end in the toes, if you prefer it this way. For instance, the first zone extends from the great toe up the entire height of the body, including the chest and the back, and down the arm into the thumb. The other digits are related to their particular zones, in like manner.

The tongue is divided into ten zones. Pressure on the dorsal (top) surface of the individual zones on the tongue affect the corresponding anterior (or front) sections of zones everywhere throughout the body. But firm pressures on the tongue, continued for several minutes, affect both back and front zones. The hard and soft palate (forming the roof of the mouth) and the posterior walls of the pharynx (the back of the throat) and epipharynx (where the back of the nose and throat join) are divided in the same way, and posterior pressure or contact affects posterior sections of zones; while anterior pressure or contact affects anterior sections of zones. Traction (or pulling with a hooked probe — see B, Fig. 11) on the soft palate in the epipharynx affects the anterior zones, and traction on the anterior pillars of the fauces, (pillars in front of the tonsils) affects zones one, two, three, four and five, especially in arms and shoulders in the posterior sections of zones. Pressure on the anterior surface of the lips and the anterior surface of the anterior pillars of the fauces affects the anterior surface of all zones. Pressure on the posterior surface of the lower lips affects the posterior sections of all zones.

Pain in any part of the first zone may be treated and overcome, temporarily at least, and often permanently, by pressure on all surfaces of the first joint of the great toe, or on the corresponding joint of the thumb. Should the pressure be limited to the upper surface of the great toe, the anesthetic or analgesic effects will extend up the front of the body to the fronto-parietal suture—where the bones join on top of the skull. They will also extend across the chest and down the anterior surface of the first zone of the arm and thumb, and often to the thumb side of the index finger. Should pressure be made on the under surface of the great toe, the effects will extend along the first zone in the sole of the foot and up the back of the leg, thigh, body and head in that zone to the above-named suture; also across the back and down the posterior surface of the first zone of the arm and thumb, and frequently the thumb side of the index finger.

Firm pressure on the end of the great toe or tip of thumb will control the entire first zone. Firm pressure on the tips of the fingers or toes control individual zones. Lateral or side pressure on thumbs and fingers or toes will affect lateral or side boundaries of the zones pressed, and also transverse extensions to nostrils, lips and ears.

A limited amount of anesthesia may often be established by pressure over any resistant bony surface, in any zone compressed, and often the mere momentary contact with the galvanic cautery, or pressure with a sharp-pointed applicator, or with the thumb or finger-nail, will produce the same result. Contacts, especially with aluminum combs or pointed instruments, may be momentary, if frequently repeated, but protracted contacts are often necessary.

Prolonged pressure with an aluminum hair comb is fast becoming a popular method, but similar pressures with the nails of the thumbs and fingers are likely the method Nature intended. Pressure with bands of elastic, metal, cloth, or leather on the fingers, toes, wrists and ankles, as well as on the knees and elbows, are often useful in overcoming pain in an individual zone or group of zones. If these pressures are resisted by pathological processes elsewhere in the zone or zones, pain is sometimes excited. In other words, if there is an abscess or some active inflammatory condition present,—as in middle-ear trouble, pressure often aggravates or stimulates the pain to renewed endeavors. It usually however, overcomes the pain momentarily. Zone pressure has, for this reason, become a diagnostic factor of great value in disclosing hidden pus conditions or inflammatory processes—particularly in the roots of teeth, the ears, appendix, ovaries, or in other organs.

Pain anywhere in any zone may be overcome more quickly by pressure with an applicator, or with cautery contact at certain points throughout the corresponding zone or zones in the mouth, pharynx, epipharynx and nose; but the finger and toe pressures may be relied upon very often. What applies to one zone applies to all.

Pressures average from one-half minute to four minutes or longer, depending upon the susceptibility of the patient.

Heat or cold waves in varying degrees, depending upon the solution or instruments used, may often be dispatched to the extremities from the mouth, nose, etc., and similar waves of heat or cold will manifest themselves in the mouth, nose and pharynx of susceptible individuals from pressure or contact on the extremities. The most susceptible patients will describe them accurately. For instance, if a cotton tipped probe be dipped in camphor solution, or alcohol, the patient will describe the sensation reflected along the particular zone pressed as "cold." If in nitrate of silver, or trichloracetic acid, he says it is "hot."

The majority of patients say that, while they are unable to detect these sensations—only extrasusceptible individuals have this faculty,—their pain is disappearing, or has already disappeared. Patients who are most susceptible to pressure or contact will trace heat or cold from an individual hair of the head, or an eyelash, to the margin of the finger-nail or toe-nail, and if a hair or eyelash be quickly pulled out, the sensation of numbness is often quickly registered beneath the finger-nail or toe-nail of the invaded zone. But

*12

to give these delicate results the subjects must be very responsive.

Pressure or contact upon the occlusal, or biting, edges of the teeth affect the innermost parts of practically every bone in the body. We believe that the teeth, being the most accessible, are the natural guardians of the bones throughout the body. The heat waves from the application of a fine point cautery contact on the biting edges of the teeth, are dispatched through the centers of all bones, and their therapeutic, or curative effect is disseminated through the bones and tissue in the zones treated. Naturally, the therapeutic effect is less marked as the surface of the body is approached.

Pressure or contact on the anterior surface of the teeth affects the anterior surface of the bones in the anterior sections of bones, and to a greater or less extent the tissues of the same zones in the corresponding sections. Pressure or contact on the posterior surface of the teeth affect the posterior surface of the bones in the posterior sections of zones treated, and to a greater or less extent the tissues of the same zones in the corresponding sections.

An asset not generally recognized in normal occlusion of a natural set of teeth is the ability of the patient to relax practically every part of the body through firm, biting pressure for two or three minutes on all surfaces of the upper and lower teeth. In this manner pain may frequently be relieved in any section of a zone, or group of zones, throughout the body, and occasionally even anesthesia may be induced through firm occlusion of the teeth for two or three minutes in these zones. This is at least one reason why all the teeth should be preserved, if at all possible, and why normal occlusion should be brought about if it does not already exist. If one be deprived of the third molar teeth, for instance, his ability to prevent, relieve or overcome pathological conditions in the fourth and fifth zones is restricted; and this naturally applies to the various individual zones or group of zones where teeth have been extracted.

You would hardly believe that offending corns or warts or bitten finger-nails, where inflammatory processes have been excited, may be responsible for rheumatism or neuritis, but we are daily proving such to be the case.

Toe-nails and finger-nails must be respected and as well taken care of, for health's sake, as any other section of the individual zones. There is not a section of a finger-nail or toe-nail that may not affect (under stimulation or pressure) the most distant parts of the body.

Also, it might be of interest here to note that while enough pressure is good, too much is mild murder. This can be testified to by all who, by means of new shoes, foolishly apply constricting pressures to their toes. There ensues, after the lapse of an appreciable length of time, a condition made up of equal parts of bodily weakness and nervous irritability—an actual physical and spiritual fatigue—relieved only by removing the pressure—in other words, by relieving zone pressure inhibition.

Tight belts, corsets, or collars will develop similar, or even worse, effects, inasmuch as their influence embraces not only the undue irritation of the nerve zones, but also the constricting influences upon glands, blood vessels and internal organs.

All zones must be free from irritation and obstructions to get the best results. For instance, if there be pain in the head, chest, abdomen, or extremities in one or more zones, it may be relieved or quite overcome by pressure on resistant surfaces anywhere in the zones affected. If the pain be relieved for a few moments only, and repeated pressures do not overcome it, it is safe to assume that the pain is due to some abnormal pressure or irritation, as gas, pus, impactions. necrosis, etc., somewhere in a zone or group of zones, which demands medical or surgical inter-ference.

We are repeatedly called upon for the theory of zone therapy. Many theories are interesting but not conclusive, and rather than be obliged to retract theories, we are not going to advance them, except very superficially, at the expense of clinical facts. It is certain that control-centers in the medulla are stimulated, as has been sug-gested, but I believe that it is shock more often than stimulation. Some theorists have pointed out, perhaps rightly, that "these functions may be carried out by the pituitary body (a ductless gland at the base of the brain) through the multiple nerve paths from it."

We know that we induce a state of inhibition —a state which prevents the transmission of the nerve impulse from the brain—throughout the zone where pressure is brought to bear. We know that when this inhibition of irritation is continuous, many pathological processes disap-pear. We are certain that lymphatic relaxation follows pressure, and the lymph stimulated to flow normally in its channels.

The theory advanced by Dr. Bowers: "that inasmuch as there are ultra-microscopic bacteria —bacteria not seen through even the highest-powered lenses,—it is more than likely that in the light of this work there are ultra-miscroscopic connections analogous to those we call nerves," may contain some elements of plausibility.

Let the physician or the dentist, who ascribes these phenomena to suggestion, attempt to relieve an aching, left-incisor, for instance, by pressing the little finger of the right hand of his patient, or exercise his persuasive powers on a throbbing molar by pressing the thumb of either hand. He will find himself up against a stone wall, so far as results are concerned, for only by exerting proper pressure, on the proper zone or zones, for an adequate length of time, will the pain disappear. Anticipating such contentions, and to avoid the merest hint at suggestion, we have purposely refrained from giving many patients any idea that we were even contemplating the relief of pain, and the first and only suggestions have been from the patient. He will tell that he experienced pain in his jaw, eye, small of back, knee, foot, or shoulder before pressure was made on his fingers, teeth, or elsewhere, and will ask, "where has the pain gone? Have you done anything to relieve it?"

Pathological conditions from irritation in the nose, epipharynx, pharynx, mouth, vagina, rectum, etc., may be responsible not only for annoying local manifestations, but for obscure pathological changes in the most remote sections of the body; and their course can usually be traced through an individual zone or group of zones. There is not an existing pathological condition that cannot at least be relieved, and a large proportion can be cured by zone therapy.

This shows how necessary it is that the physician and surgeon should be capable of diagnosing and treating disease in all parts of the body, especially if his practice be limited to the country, where he may be unable to consult with specialists. If the pathological condition he has treated does not "clear up," the case should be referred to the specialist or dentists, for, to secure results, all parts of the zones or group of zones must be free from obstruction and irritation.

Zone therapy demonstrates the co-relation of all parts of the body, also the manner in which pressure or contact upon certain zones is effective in the relief of pain or disease.

Diagnosis of the cause of pain may be worked out quite perfectly over or through any zone or part of zone. If a patient complains of pain, and indicates that the right eye is involved, and you overcome the pain by pressure on the front of the right index finger, it is absolutely certain that his disturbance is excited by congestion or irritation in the anterior section of the zone; but if it be necessary to look to the palmar surface of the index finger for relief the cause is certain to exist in the posterior section of the zone or zones.

We have never suggested this work as a panacea, but finding it helpful in the treatment of human ills, we consider it an asset to our knowledge of medicine and surgery, and have been glad to offer it gratuitously to physicians, surgeons, and dentists, and to all who can make use of it in the relief of afflicted humanity.

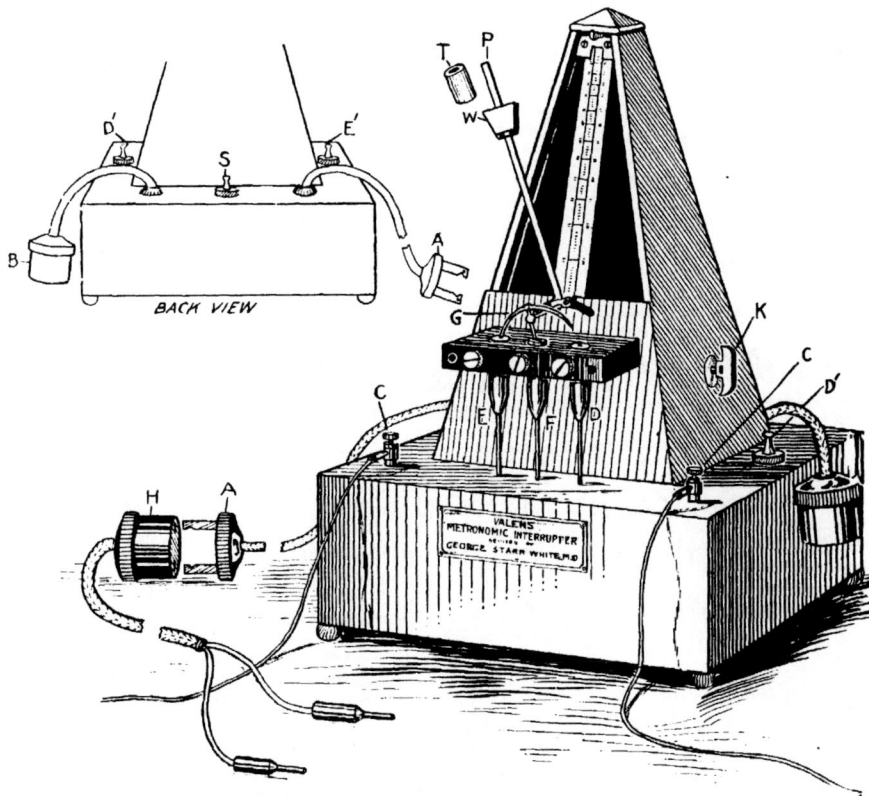

Valens Metronomic Interrupter (Style D)
(For Producing Dr. White's Pulsoidal Current)

FIG. 33.

CHAPTER 18.

FOOD FOR THOUGHT.

WHEN "Professor" Robert Fitzsimmons delivered the famous punch in the solar plexus that laid the mighty James Corbett upon whatever it is they cover a boxing ring with, he demonstrated to everybody's satisfaction—except perhaps Mr. Corbett's—that there is a group of nerves in the "pit of the stomach" which has an intimate and most distressful connection with the brain. And now every doctor knows the functions and connections of the pneumogastric nerve.

Gunmen, pugilists, and "bouncers" also know that if the temple, or the angle of the jaw, be even lightly "tapped," the tappee is usually placed hors de combat for an appreciable period of time. General knowledge of this weighty academic subject is comparatively recent—as time is reckoned.

And the Japs, in their uncanny knowledge of nerve anatomy, exemplified in their proficiency in jui jitsu, have shown that, by pressure upon certain nerve terminals, or upon plexuses of

(186)

nerve groups they are able to do almost every-
thing except murder a victim. Perhaps they
could do this, also, if they were sufficiently in-
dustrious and persevering.

Indeed, for many years they have been aware
that there are certain nerve centers in the neck
and under the angle of the jaw, pressure upon
which will temporarily suspend consciousness.
In fact, their methods were tried by surgeons,
prior to the discovery of anesthesia; but were
discarded, owing to the fact that no one could
guarantee that the patients would wake again
after the operation.

Also, as showing how great oaks from little
acorns grow, and how mickle and mickle makes
muckle, Professor William Halstead, more than
a dozen years ago, was operating upon a man
with a rupture—under cocaine anesthesia, as he
thought. It was found, however, after the operation had been painlessly completed, that the
moon-stricken assistant had forgotten to put the
cocaine tablet in the syringe.

So that all the anesthetic the patient got was
sterile water. However, this was enough, for
the pressure of the water injection into the parts,
had blocked the nerve tract, and inhibited the
transmission of the message of pain.

This experience may or may not have given

Dr. Crile the clue to his interesting and vastly important discovery of "nerve block," but, in any event, we learned something new about the human body. But—and this is the point I wish to emphasize — we are not through learning about it yet.

So, if some time a doctor tells you that a woman of sixty-nine, suffering for years from one-sided paralysis, made pressures twice daily with an aluminum comb on the top (or front) of the hand, favoring the thumb side—and in two weeks noticed a decided improvement, and after five months can now lift her foot free from the floor and walk without a cane, don't sneer.

If another tells you that a case of infantile paralysis, of five years' standing—after several months' treatment with a probe on the back wall of the pharynx, can now kick as high as his shoulder with either foot, don't scoff. For that doctor has photos of the boy, showing him in the act of doing just this identical thing.

It may also be that catarrhal appendicitis is helped. For in unorthodox ways three cases of catarrhal appendicitis were apparently cured by pressures exerted with a comb over the first, second and third finger, and carried up as far as the wrist. These cases were diagnosed as catarrhal appendicitis by several competent medical men. They showed all the classical symptoms, including pain on pressure over Mc-Burney's point, vomiting, and digestive disturbances. They were treated three times daily for several days, and in the interim, treated themselves at home along the same lines. In ten days to two weeks, there was an apparent cure of all three cases. And now, after six months, there has been no return of the condition.

And, speaking of appendicitis, it is interesting to note that if pain is relieved by zone pressure, and returns after a short time, we can be morally certain that there is pus present, and that the case demands immediate operation. This same thing, as we before observed, applies to abscesses in the ear, teeth, tonsil, or anywhere else.

The injunction to "prove all things and hold fast to that which is true," is as applicable and pertinent today as it was when first dropped from the lips of the old sage. So, if some time your progressive doctor should tell you to rub your finger nails together, and scratch the front of your hands and arms, and thereby cure falling hair, don't laugh—because he may be repeating to you only what numbers of his patients have told him they did—and stopped their hair from leaving its moorings.

Also, if he tells you to use a wire brush on the

front and back of the hand, and also press with
the aluminum comb on the palms of the hand, to
cure cold feet, he may not be nearly as crazy as
he sounds. He may be merely a little ahead of
your time, as were Harvey, Semmelweis, Horace
Wells, Lister, and hundreds of others, who have
suffered the slings and arrows of ridicule.

And so, we who believe in zone therapy now
understand why we grind our teeth. It is because the action relieves nerve tension, and
diminishes the pain in all the zones of the body
connected by those invisible and as yet undis-
covered nervous wires strung through the telegraph poles of the teeth.

When we grab our bruised shins we check the
transmission of pain in the irritated nerve trunk
lines of that zone. When we grasp the arm of
the dental chair, and hang on like grim death,
we are unconsciously going through motions
that, if continued long enough, would have made
our trial comparatively painless. The only fault
in our preparation for the ordeal was that we
should have started our pressure grip three or
four minutes earlier. But our intentions were
good.

When automatically we clench our fists in
furious anger, we are relieving our terrific
nervous excitation, and thereby perhaps pre-

venting the bursting of a blood vessel. When we clasp the hands of one sorely stricken and in the throes of despair, we are, in addition to supplying him with comforting magnetism and physical solace, producing a distinctly analgesic and quieting effect upon his entire nervous system.

And when we clasp our hands or press the fingers tightly together in supplication, we are ministering to over-wrought nerves, and thereby perhaps bringing ourselves into closer harmony with the great Cosmic Force that envelopes us all in a mantle of kindness and love.

[CONCLUSION.]

Printed in the United States
34239LVS00005B/253